Vegan Sex

By Ellen Jaffe Jones

Recipes By Beverly Lynn Bennett

Contributor Joel K. Kahn MD.

To Lisa D. —
Hope you get inspired!
Ellen Jaffe Jones

Published by Vegcoach Publishing

First edition May 2017

By Ellen Jaffe Jones

Vegan Coach, Vegan Mythbusting Queen,
Bestselling Author, Radio Co-Host,
Certified Personal Trainer (AFAA) and Running Coach

Recipes By Beverly Lynn Bennett
Vegan Chef and Bestselling Author

By Joel K. Kahn MD
Top Doc/Cardiologist and #1 Bestselling Author

Inside you will find over
100 Delicious Recipes
you can begin making TODAY!

Warning:

This book has already proven to be controversial within the vegan community. Sex
and sexuality is part of our everyday life. The failure of healthy sex, known as erectile
dysfunction, is the #1 leading indicator by a few months or a few decades of killer heart
attacks and heart disease...all which can be avoided with a whole foods plant-based diet.
Having a respected cardiologist, such as Dr. Joel Kahn, partner on this book not only
begins conversations that should be happening, but provides sound information from a
practicing and respected vegan doctor who is saving lives with diet.

Dedicated to my daughters, Rebecca, Jessica and Aron. Our children's future prospects for a healthy life and planet hang in the balance of whether we get global warming, climate change and the fate of human and non-human health right as soon as possible.

And to my parents who were so sick and diseased they couldn't lift my babies, let alone babysit them. Entire generations are losing each other and don't even know it. Preventable pain and suffering should not exist anywhere, not in this day and age.

Table of Contents

Dedication iii

Endorsements 13

Acknowledgements 17

Introduction 23

Chapter 1   Who Woulda Thunk? Erectile Dysfunction is the
             Canary in the Coal Mine--The Leading Indicator of
             Heart Disease and More 29

Chapter 2   Invading Privacy to Tell the Truth 41

Dr Joel Kahn M.D. contributed Chapters 3-5
Chapter 3   The Research on Heart Disease and What It Means
             to Erectile Dysfunction: Of Hard Attacks and
             Heart Attacks: Why Should a Cardiologist Care? 73

Chapter 4   The Physiology of Sex and Food: Vegans,
             Vaginas, Vegetables and Vas Deferens 81

Chapter 5   Plants and Herbs in Your Pants 93

Chapter 6   The Epiphany: Mind-blowing Differences Between
             Vegan and Non-Vegan Sex.. 99

Chapter 7   If Sex is 95% Between the Ears,
             Why Being Vegan Matters 127

Chapter 8   The Weirdest Thing That Ever Happened or
             the World's Worst (Almost) Vegan Date 133

Chapter 9   The Male Perspective: Why You Might Want
             to Pay Attention if You're a Guy............................. 149

Chapter 10   How a Vegan Diet Affects Women and Sex:
             A Personal Story 155

Chapter 11   Getting Real Personal: Why Vegans Do It Better 161

Chapter 12   Vegan Aphrodisiacs--Why Is This A Thing? 169

Chapter 13   Exercises to Spice It Up 181

Chapter 14   Resources for Vegan Singles and Couples.................... 195

Chapter 15   Vegan Sex Toys and Products–
             Being Mission Consistent................................. 199

Vegan Sex Recipes.. 209

Beverly Lynn Bennett contributed all of the below recipes
Chapter 16   Morning Quickies--Quick Beverages
             and Morning Options.. 211

             -   Chai Tea for Two.. 212
             -   Mango Lassi 213
             -   Arousing Avocado Green Smoothie 214
             -   Hot Bahama Mama Smoothie 215
             -   Dutch Apple Pie Smoothie............................. 216
             -   Mexican Hot Chocolate Smoothie 217
             -   Ambrosia.. 218
             -   Passion Fruit Breakfast Bowls......................... 219
             -   Pistachio, Dried Fruit, and Yogurt Delight................. 220

- Good Morning Muesli..221
- Grab Bag Granola...222
- Strawberry and Cashew Cream Cheese Spread.............224
- Avocado Toast with Coconut Bacon 225
- Fruit-n-Nut Rice Cakes 227

Chapter 17 Lingering Breakfasts (or Brunches) in
Bed--Breakfast/Brunch Options and Baked Goods 229
- Rum Banana Roll Ups 230
- Vanilla-Almond French Toast 232
- Berry Nice and Spice Pancakes...................................233
- Baked Latkes with Applesauce 235
- Tempeh Bacon...237
- Seitan Sausages 238
- No Eggs Scramble with Chiles and Greens 240
- Herb and Cheese Biscuits..241
- Raspberry, Chocolate Chip, and Yogurt Scones...........243
- Banana Bread 245
- Carrot Cake Muffins 246
- Cappuccino-Chip Muffins 247

Chapter 18 Afternoon Delights--Soups, Salads, and Sandwiches 249
- Gingery Carrot Soup...250
- Mexican Tortilla Soup 251
- Mood-Enhancing Mushroom Soup............................252
- White Bean Chili...253
- Pho You Noodle Bowls...254
- Avocado, Fennel, and Citrus Salad 255
- Greek-Style Chickpea Salad 256
- Aphrodite Salad with Pomegranate Dressing...............257
- Cleopatra Salad with Hemp Seed Dressing..................258
- Pacific Northwest Kale Salad 259
- Avocado Dream Spread...260

- Black Bean and Mango Salad Lettuce Wraps.................261
- Italian-Style Vegetable Hoagies.............................262
- Chocolate-Nut Butter Spread and Banana Paninis.......263
- Baked Falafel and Cucumber Tzatziki
  Pita Sandwiches...265
- Quarter Pounder Beet Burgers 267

Chapter 19 Naughty Nibbles--Snacks and Appetizers.......................271

- Bliss Balls...272
- Apricot Delights...273
- Cinnamon and Vanilla-Kissed Almonds....................275
- Cocoa-Coated Cashews.......................................276
- Sweet and Savory Snack Mix 277
- Santa Fe Trail Mix..278
- Lemon-Herb Roasted Chickpeas 280
- Fruit-n-Nut Crackers...281
- Artichoke Pâté 283
- Kalamata Olive Hummus.....................................284
- Whoo-Pea Guacamole with Baked Tortilla Chips........285
- Papaya-Pineapple Salsa 287
- Smoked Cheddar Cashew Cheese Ball 288
- Hot Artichoke and Spinach Dip............................289
- Cucumber Canapés with Red Pepper Spread...............291
- Crispy Buffalo Cauliflower with Ranch Dressing..........292

Chapter 20 A Little Something on the Side--Side Dishes 295

- Citrus-Scented Asparagus....................................296
- Lemon and Ginger-Infused Steamed Vegetables..........297
- Steamed Artichokes with Creamy Saffron-Almond
  Dipping Sauce...299
- Roman-Style Artichoke and Asparagus Bake.............301
- Broccoli and Cheese-Topped Baked Potatoes.............302
- Ginger and Coconut Water-Braised Carrots.................304

- Spiced and Smashed Sweet Potatoes..............................305
- Bayou Beans..306
- Okra Soycatash...308
- Roasted Roots...309
- Tomatoes Rockefeller..311
- Pistachio and Grape-Studded Quinoa.........................313
- Orange-Scented Couscous with Apricots,
  Cherries, and Pine Nuts 315
- Confetti Coconut Basmati Rice 316
- Down-n-Dirty Rice...317
- Farro with Lacinato Kale and Pomegranate Seeds........319

Chapter 21 Main Events--Main Dishes..321
- Mushroom and Veggie Fajitas...................................322
- Green Gumbo...323
- Veggie Paella..325
- Sweet and Sour Tofu and Vegetables.........................326
- Pesto-Swirled Polenta...328
- Bacon Cheeseburger Mac-n-Cheese..........................330
- Pasta Primavera..332
- Pasta Puttanesca...334
- Pita Pizza Party..336
- BBQ Seitan Strips..337
- Winter Squash with Apple-Walnut Stuffing 339
- Supper-Sized Stuffed Florentine Portobellos..............341
- Cornmeal and Pumpkin Seed Breaded Tempeh..........343
- Coconut-Crusted Cutlets with Sweet
  Thai Chili Sauce..345
- Hot Tamale Pie...347

Chapter 22 Happy Endings--Sweet Treats and Desserts....................351
- Raw Fruit Delights 352
- Spiked Dark Chocolate Truffles 353

- Cherry Amaretto Chia Seed Pudding 355
- Amazing Avocado-Chocolate Mousse 356
- Filled Figs Three Way 357
- Vanilla-Infused Banana Ice Cream and Partners 359
- Whipped Coconut Cream 360
- After Dark Chocolate Sauce and Fondue-for-Two 361
- Cherries Jubilee 363
- Mulled Wine Poached Pears 365
- Sugar-n-Spice-Kissed Cookies 367
- Making Whoopie Pies 369
- Vegan Berry Cheesecake 371
- Vanilla Pound Cake 373
- Devil's Food Cake with After Dark Ganache 375

Eating vegan can sometimes
be challenging -

We wrote this book not only to
provide facts, but also to help
you along your journey when it
comes to a thriving, healthy lifestyle,
inside and outside of the bedroom.

We are here for you:
Ellen Jaffe Jones - www.vegcoach.com
Beverly Lynn Bennett - www.veganchef.com
Joel K. Kahn M.D. - www.drjoelkahn.com

Endorsements

"The way of eating that's been shown to reverse heart disease and type 2 diabetes, improve recovery for athletes and make weight lost last, now has an even sexier benefit: better sex! Going vegan has always been about love for all life, and this book shows that it's just what the doctor - and his champion-athlete coauthor - ordered for your love life too."

- Victoria Moran, author of Main Street Vegan
and director of Main Street Vegan Academy

"The only thing better than a good morning is a wood morning!! ED has been called ground zero of cardiovascular disease. A morning erection can serve as a daily systems check that should put a smile on your face...and maybe even your partner's "

- Marco Borges author NYT Bestseller The 22 Days Revolution
and founder of 22 Days Nutrition

"The adult human has about 100,000 miles of blood vessels. With our typical American diet, we damage and block them. Our health goes to waste for short-term taste. This book will instruct you how to improve blood vessel function and return to the nature we were meant to have. Let's change our lifestyles and really enjoy our lives."

- Kim Allan William, Sr. M.D., James B. Herrick Professor Chief,
Division of Cardiology
Rush University Medical Center, Chicago

"The same diet that closes the arteries to the heart and brain has the same effect on other arteries - and often arterial function decline shows up first in organs other than the heart. Isn't it time we bring this behind-closed-doors conversation out into the light of day? Vegan Sex has done an enlightening, provocative, and entertaining job of doing just that."

- Lani Muelrath, Amazon best-selling author
of The Plant-Based Journey, Fit Quickies, and The Mindful Vegan

"Healthy eating can add more than just years to your life, but life to your years—healthy people have more fun! Read this book to learn how."

- Michael Greger, M.D. FACLM
of NutritionFacts.org, author of How Not to Die

"great subject, great book"

- Russell Simmons

"Among the many surprises of a healthy plant-based diet is—yes—better sex. It's not just that the diet makes you a more attractive partner with better skin and a trimmer waistline. It actually improves blood flow where it counts and gets your hormones back into balance.

"Vegan Sex is a an eye-opening, jaw-dropping guide to everything you never knew about sex and how to get your body back in action. Proven by research studies and personal experience, and written in an engaging—sometimes irreverent—style, this simple method works better than a wheelbarrow full of Viagra."

- Neal D. Barnard, MD, FACC, Adjunct Associate Professor of Medicine, George Washington University School of Medicine President, Physicians Committee

Acknowledgements

So many people contributed to this book, knowingly or not. First, to the amazing Dr. Joel Kahn, otherwise humbly known on social media and elsewhere as "America's Healthy Heart Doc." It was a rainy, raw day in Ft. Myers, Florida where Dr. Kahn was headed my way, and I was unloading a trunk full of books getting ready for the South Florida Vegfest, where we were both speakers. I saw his shirt that loudly said, "Vegan is Sexy" which prompted me to say half joking, "Ya know, I'm writing a book called 'Vegan Sex.' Want to co-author?" My publisher turned down my proposal (the only one they've ever nixed) saying they needed a cardiologist's point of view. Dr. Kahn immediately and kindly said yes, and in less than an hour, during his talk at Vegfest, he announced from the stage, our plans to co-author. I was delighted that he was a person like me, trying to put dreams into action faster than the speed of light. He has been a welcome addition. Of course, given that a vegan diet is optimal for saving lives and the planet, many of us believe we should have been vegan yesterday. Under that umbrella, perhaps it makes sense why so many of us are energetic and eager to get our messages heard in a world that is dominated by pay-to-play corporate agendas.

With a cardiologist on board, I thought my publisher would jump at the opportunity. But they still said no, thinking that the concept of vegan sex wouldn't sell. I love my publisher, and have other deals in the works. I thought it took wonderful grace to say, "We might be wrong on this."

With all due respect, I disagree, which is why I decided to self-publish for the first time. I totally believe, as many others do, that if the world knew how ah-MA-zing a vegan diet is for sexual performance and long-lasting relationships in and out of bed, the conversion rate of carnivores to vegans would be through the roof. Dr. Kahn shared my belief and vision, and I was excited to have him especially as a cardiologist, on board. The cardiologists really do get the vegan "thang." Continuing ed on a vegan diet and its effect on heart disease continue to swell in attendance for doctors.

A big thanks to one of my publisher's superstar recipe developers and authors, Beverly Lynn Bennett. We burned the midnight oil at Chicago's Veggiefest, and after sharing my book idea with her, she asked if she could write recipes that showcase some of the best vegan aphrodisiacs. You're going to love her contributions. Plus, she's been loving and having fabulous vegan sex with the same vegan guy for 30 years.

I hope that sharing my stories, some of them very painful, will help you in your decision to go and stay vegan. If you're new to the vegan table, the word means not eating, using, buying or exploiting anything with a mother or a face. No animal use whatsoever.

Sometimes life is the best teacher. If my mistakes help others in their choices, then it is all worth it. Others contributed to this book with their stories, experience and knowledge. They chose or I opted to keep them anonymous, even in the acknowledgements and understandably so. Some of their stories were painful to share too, even though their sharing was only with me. I appreciate their courage and candor. You know who you are.

The list of those OK with a thank you here includes but is not limited to Gabrielle Lennon, Reggie Adams, Jonathan Balcombe, Miyoko Schinner,

Steve Blumberg, Bob and Cynthia Holzapfel, David Kidd, Rebecca Gilbert, Alan Roettinger, Trevor Chin, Rebecca Gilbert, everyone in Florida Voices for Animals and animal and vegan activists everywhere, plus a slew of too many littered relationships which shall remain in the pyre of life's unnamed failures. Failures can be our greatest teachers.

To the courageous vegan doctors and dieticians who have risked their reputation and livelihoods, swimming upstream and going against conventional wisdom and medicine to truly do no harm. They should all win Nobel Prizes for following their consciences on what is in the best interests of patients and clients.

My fav doctors along with the nonprofits and organizations they run include Drs. John McDougall, Neal Barnard, Joel Fuhrman, T. Colin Campbell, Michael Greger, Michael Klaper, Caldwell Esselstyn, Baxter Montgomery, Terry Mason, Garth Davis, Heather Shenkman, Milton Mills and Alan Goldhammer. These names often appear consistently on the top 10 lists of vegan doctors. Some have been around for decades modestly promoting the message of vegan health. Other younger doctors have seen how well this good vegan medicine works on patients, often way better than drugs. Some have written their own books and are doing what they can to get the message out.

As people like me and so many others have spread the success and recovery to good health after having read their books, their popularity, finally in due course, has soared. If you haven't, go right out and read their books. My publisher tells his authors, "It takes decades to be an overnight success." As the popularity and powerful effects of a vegan diet grow, people are discovering that a healthful version of vegan eating happily fuels someone like me who can race and place in lots of running races while watching everybody in her family succumb to disease. I had fibrocystic breast disease, many benign tumors removed all over my body, and almost died of a colon blockage. I didn't get all the good genes. As I sometimes joke to hide the pain, I may come from the sickest family in America.

I wish more women and doctors of color were on this doctor list, but it is what it is. While the percentage of women doctors has grown from 9.7 percent in in 1970 to 32.4 percent in 2010, the abysmal representation is sad. More depressing is that recent figures show a trend that enrollment by women in medical school is declining.

As the popularity of veganism rises, so do the mounting voices of dissent, some even calling the hero doctors charlatans and hucksters conniving to take your money. Nothing could be farther from the truth. Make no mistake. Their courageous work saves lives daily. Testimonials abound online everywhere to support that, including my own recovery from almost dying of that colon blockage, at age 28.

A special thanks to my dear friend, Jen Kaden, who has done so much to help organize the Cleveland Vegfest, one of the best and biggest in the US. She has been a great mentor in her organizational and human relations skills. Understanding the opposite sex is never easy.

And finally, to my special friend, Val McDaniel, one of the most thoughtful and giving people I've ever met. Asking, "What can I do today to make you happy?" along with initiating many random acts of kindness for me, casual acquaintances and even strangers, has been something I wasn't used to and didn't think was possible in a very cranky mixed up world. His editing skills were also invaluable. In recent times, he has been at every race I've done, and every vegan event to offer support and encouragement. His voice, the loudest at all races, yelling "Go Ellen," in addition to any other runner whose name he knows, keeps me motivated and focused on the toughest of days. He noticed all kinds of changes as he went vegan in and out of bed, and watching his transformation from smoking, steak and potatoes was one of the main inspirations for this book. I realized the impact of his change when his daughter gave him a handmade shirt that said, on the front, "What Happens When You Eat Vegan?" The underside of the shirt flipped up and said, "She Moans." I'll let you interpret that however you like. He also provided many yucks to my co-authors and me by Googling, "Vegetables that Look Like Sex Organs." We had no idea. We will never look at oranges and radishes the same way again.

Warning...this is a bit of an X-rated book. By definition, it has to be. My co-authors shared many jokes and puns along the way, too. I'm sure you'll develop your own humor, once you realize how much better for yourself, your partner, the planet and the animals vegan sex can be. You may even wonder like me, after being so shocked and even outraged at the differences between vegan and non-vegan sex, why did it take me so long?

Introduction

Vegans do it better. They just do. It's all about blood flow. If I had to boil this book down to a few sentences, those statements would nail it. But alas, it isn't always that easy or black and white. This book will tell you how and why. I was a vegan virgin. If you haven't had sex with a vegan, you're a vegan virgin too.

I come up with ideas for books in some pretty far-reaching places in my brain. If there is a theme, it is consistent with the radio show I've hosted over the years, "The Vegan Mythbusters." Misinformation and disinformation play out in harder to recognize faux or "alt" news. Not a day or a social media page goes by without some outrageous, outlandish assumption or fact error, or "alternative fact" about living as a vegan.

Mission in life: to blow up every vegan myth. Mission in this book: to let you know how easy and fun it is to live your life as a vegan…in and out of bed. It's not some misguided, crazy activist gone off the deep end theory. This is based in science, facts, a lifetime of experiences and yes finally, a passionate activist who just can't stand the falsehoods promoted on a daily basis by those who are guided by meat and dairy corporate interests.

This book, like most, was born in the "write what you know" department and erupted in a time when I thought, what if it's really true, peace begins with me, at home. Clean up your own house first. I've been through a few marriages and relationships, to put it mildly. Is it possible, I've honestly asked myself, that my partners and I weren't satisfied and therein began the problems? Were their feelings associated with "failure to perform" not in the mind at all, but mostly or totally in the body exclusively? Was the sexual inadequacy of my partners responsible for their thoughts of not feeling they were good enough? My partners were heavy meat and dairy eaters before I went vegan, for sure. After I went vegan, they would say that they ate a healthy diet, but in all cases, they still consumed, even on occasion, fish and/or dairy.

All of this, including the suicide of one partner made me dig deep. While I know that a vegan diet is not a guarantee against so many diseases and conditions, it can help many others. I wondered, did my partners transfer their own feelings of inadequacy to criticism of me? How much did an animal-heavy diet block their arteries, including those in the brain? Did erectile dysfunction make them suspicious, constantly accusatory for no valid reason, and eventually nasty and violent? Was ED truly at the root of our worst problems? If more men knew how virile, strong and long-lasting they could be eating a vegan diet, would we not have more vegan men? I think you know the answer to that. And we would have a whole lot more happy women.

I am as biased as a reporter can be on this topic. Many of my partners who suffered from ED seemed quite clear: they blamed it on deep-seated psychological feelings of inadequacies. But what if that wasn't entirely true, or true at all? What if their ED was purely or mostly physical in nature, and instead of a pill that caused all kinds of side-effects, some known, perhaps some not, they changed their diet?

My reporter's righteous indignation began erupting and asking: With the physical changes almost immediate, how many relationships could be saved? How many blame games could end and relationships revived? What if ED was pretty much a physical condition and not emotionally caused, as so many people believe? What if it wasn't the psychological self-fulling prophecy that so many think it is?

I probably can't get away with 100% of the blame going outward. It always takes two to tango. But deep-seated inadequacies about sexual performance are well-documented in our Type A, get it first and get it right culture. Not to sound too out there, but I've long been complimented on my patience, kindness and perseverance in personality and also when it comes to pleasing men, both emotionally and physically. Like many women, I spent years in therapy alone, and then eventually with partners exploring "what did I do wrong?" One ED-afflicted ex told me I was too emotional and needed to think more rationally, like him. Did he just not get that this is often how the two sexes split the division of emotional labor? Or, in my passion to give as much as I could to the world, or enthusiasm to live life to the fullest, did I expect too much and forget to take my theoretical chill pill? Of course, many women tend to believe there is something wrong with them when their man is not happy. They run to the therapist first trying to fix what they think is broken from within, justifiably so, or perhaps not.

As I began to spread the word I was writing this book more than two years ago, almost everyone I mentioned it to greeted the concepts and ideas enthusiastically, greeting me with eyes widened, giggles and nodding in agreement that I was truly on to something. Certainly, I have lived both sides of this coin, have cried way too many tears trying to figure out how to make it work, "it" being the relationship. Finally, arriving in my current relationship, I was greeted by someone who was not vegan but saw the benefits big time, and supported me in ways I had only dreamed about. He finds new and different ways to support me, and every so often asks, "How have you not had anyone who has supported you this way?" Indeed, I wonder that too, but am grateful for however it plays out. After this last experience, there is no doubt in my mind that if my exes had changed to a vegan diet, they would have enjoyed a satisfying sex life, and would not have the designation of "ex" in my life. I knew something was wrong...the constant fighting, the cantankerousness, the edginess, the combativeness, all a part, I believe, the direct result of not getting much satisfaction physically and emotionally. In addition, as Dr. Neal Barnard points out, there is too much testosterone from an animal-heavy diet that plays out in road rage every day. But with clogged arteries, the excess hormones have nowhere to go. Is healthy sex that important? Yes. Absolutely!

When I wrote the book, "Kitchen Divided," it was the direct result of living with husbands up to that point who were not vegan. As I toured the country speaking about my first book, "Eat Vegan on $4 a Day," as an aside, I once asked my audience, "So how many of you live in 'mixed marriages,' where one of you is veg and the other is not?" With much laughter, consternation and rolling of eyes into backs of heads, hands shot up like wildfires. I began asking the question repeatedly, and knew I was on to something. In my travels and in many of the stories people shared with me, I know that there are tons of vegans who are able to live in mixed marriages successfully.

But I look back on my writing of that book and realize it was nothing more than a huge justification of my budding dissatisfaction with my ex's resentment and anger of my growing success with my vegan books and speeches around the US. I had put up with his eating Spam and buying his deli meat long enough. I stood by his side when he had his heart attack. I was there 30 days in the cardiac rehab unit to the tune of a million dollars of Medicare money, the nurses said. When he woke up from his bi-pass surgery and said, "I never want to feel this pain again, help me go vegan," I was hopeful. So hopeful. It lasted a month. While my patience was waning, I still hung in there, believing in that "till death do us part," mantra. However, I would shortly realize it wasn't going to be my death. Without spelling out the specifics, if you Google symptoms and conditions leading up to heart disease, oxygen deprivation and apnea, these are the most common symptoms. As a result, delusions set in, and they can become violent. I'll just leave it at that and say that I gave it my best shot. Everyone has to draw their line in the sand and determine when enough is enough. Personal safety is right up at the top for most of us, no matter how much we may love or had loved our partners. It was not an easy or quick decision.

Partnerships can be good in humans as we nurture, care, and grow with each other. Or in some cases, as in my own, they're good for driving one's ex to the hospital while he was having an active heart attack. Our relationship eventually ended mainly due to his not respecting my veganism and more. Yes, there's always more as we realize we never know a person until we go through some of life's toughest challenges. As my father trying to instill values of compassion advised me, "You never know what goes on behind closed doors."

The increasing hostility my ex developed over my veganism became painfully and embarrassingly evident and visible in public. That, coupled with threatened violence was my main ticket out. The day we eventually split, he told me his therapist made him thank me, giving me credit for saving his life after hospital personnel pointed that he came within an hour of dying. Forgiveness is such a thing now. If it helps him leave this world with a clearer conscience, a big whatever.

Point being, especially as we age, it's always good to have a partner who is at least physically around. Many people don't consider the side effects of various diseases. Some of those side effects are well-known and discussed. Others are not. It's important to know what you are getting yourself into if you choose a partner who is not vegan, shows no interest in it and has some or many of the diseases of affluence such as diabetes, heart disease, cancer and more. For the growing masses of people who choose to live alone, there are always EMS devices for notifying first responders.

So that was my final epiphany. After going through hell and back, I vowed I would never again live with anyone who wasn't vegan. While many vegans can and do live with and among non-vegans, it is important to understand some of the more dire end-of-life consequences and health disasters that can occur physically, emotionally and especially financially. I won't go there too much on that last one other than to say, two can live more cheaply than one, and divorce at an older age (at any age really, but especially in the senior years) can be incredibly complicated and devastating.

Some might say that we are using sex and guilt to sell this book first and veganism second. What we want to make clear is selling good health at a low cost is our priority. Healthy, long-lasting sex is often a side-effect of a healthy heart and other plant-fueled organs and bodies. Failed sex is often the leading indicator, by a decade or two, of more serious diseases about to come. Not in every case, but very often, it is an early warning signal to redirect your choices and your life, before a heart attack kills you. Genes do not determine destiny. There's much you can do to change your fate.

I wish for you nothing but good karma, bliss and joy in your relationships. But if mama told you life was always going to be a bowl of cherries, she was lying. To the extent you can benefit from my mistakes and experiences, I open my heart widely. No one should experience the preventable physical and emotional pain and suffering I've seen in my life. No one. We know too much from the courageous vegan hero doctors and dieticians who have shared their knowledge and time with the world for several decades now. We are the lucky ones to benefit from them and redo and reboot our lives accordingly. If you are lucky enough to find a partner who gets it and gets you, count your blessings every day. If not, you might find some interesting tools in these pages to begin your recruitment today. Knowledge is power.

In good health in and out of bed!

Ellen Jaffe Jones–Vegan Mythbuster!

CHAPTER 1

Who Woulda Thunk?
Erectile Dysfunction is the Canary in the Coal Mine–The Leading Indicator of Heart Disease and More

When I first came up with the concept for this book, some of my vegan women friends adamantly went, "Nope, not so fast. My husband is vegan and has erectile dysfunction." But my sense from research and experience is that the odds of not having ED are much better for vegans.

I was asked, "How do you feel about sharing some of these really private and painful experiences?" Here's why I'm so willing to put myself out there and be passionate and outspoken for this hush-hush issue that not many are willing to come forward and speak about. If it helps others avoid preventable suffering, then it is totally worth it. Erectile dysfunction, and it's cause, artery disease, is a huge elephant in the room. While it isn't always the case, more often than not it is---it's all about blood flow. Simply, erectile dysfunction is the canary in the coal mine. Dr. Kahn shares the detailed medical description of this analogy. In lay terms, so to speak, it is the leading indicator of heart disease. Where there's smoke, there's fire. But way more than the leading indicator of disease, the physical inadequacies of our bodies play out in huge emotional and psychological ways we are only just beginning to understand. Many mainstream doctors have no reservations telling their patients with ED that it is the leading indicator of heart disease. Vegan doctors have been screaming it from the rooftops for decades.

Simply, I've had sexual experiences with both vegans and non-vegans. The contrast for me was stark. Astounding! I had never had sex with a vegan until my 60's. It blew me away. It just blew me away. We'll get into the whys in a little. And I'll just say at the top here...no, I'm not giving any specifics. Not saying who, how, or when. So don't even ask. Ever. ;) These details really aren't important. Protecting privacy, however, is more important.

Most importantly, I was stunned by the difference. I was elated not to face deflated issues, so to speak. Joyful and happy. Then I got angry. It was the same feeling I had when I realized and saw how by going on a vegan diet years ago, I could reduce my cholesterol, avoid lifelong constipation, heart disease, diabetes and obesity that destroyed my family and friends. What if none of my exes and men I'd known never had erectile dysfunction? What differences would it have made? I can only begin to ponder that question, as you must too.

Remember the joy you felt when you first went vegan? At first you were so ecstatic, and then you got angry as you wondered why no doctor shared this lifesaving information with you before. I truly believe knowing the truth about how sex is impacted by diet would have made all the difference in the world for so many reasons which we will explore.

The anger I experienced was similar to when I almost died of a colon blockage at the age of 28. When I learned how the worst pain of my life (and the lives of millions of other victims of this easily preventable condition) could have been completely avoided, I was infuriated. I was incensed that lifelong, painful constipation, to the point of a pediatrician making house calls for such pains when I was 5 years old, was reversed in a few meals. Permanently. What is wrong with medical education that doctors don't "prescribe" a high fiber, whole foods diet as a first line of defense or remedy, instead of a smorgasbord of drugs?

As for sexual function, I was angry that nobody in the mainstream or traditional health care system shared the love, in part, because they never got a nutrition class in medical school. I was angry that my sexual partners, like me, were clueless about the link between diet and fine sex.

One more thing. Between marriages and significant and not so significant others, I don't want to identify any of them. So when I use the word "ex," it means one of them. Again, not naming names.

We study and taste fine wine in all kinds of educational settings. Why did sex get left on the back burner? How many marriages could have been saved with some mighty fine sex to smooth over the ruffles of everyday ho-hum and tumultuous living in a crazy and getting crazier world?

Yeah, yeah, sex isn't everything. For someone who's reasonably smart, I always gave lip-service to wanting guys to like me for my heart and brains. Once I began working in television news, looks became even more of a focal point, especially as I aged. I knew that at the age of 40, the handwriting was on the wall. Even though I looked younger than most people my age back then, the TV make-up consultant said 40 was never too young to have a facelift, and the more often I had them at a younger age, the more effective they would be long term. She pointed out, both male and female, who had had them. She mentioned them by names, at the local and national level, concluding with the line I'll never forget, "You don't get to be Barbara Walters' age and look like that."

While having an OK body can help with initial attraction and interest, I always wanted the focus to be away from looks. I wanted to like my partners for their kindness, compassion, empathy, smarts and big hearts. I hoped it would work the same way in return. But as I would learn, the physical side and emotional intimacy can go a long way to bridge the chasms, disagreements and differences between the sexes. And even more, the heart-mind connection is intricately interwoven between the expression of sexuality. That's the 95% between the ears part.

Don't mess with a former Emmy-winning TV investigative reporter, or at least reporters who are trained at schools where ethics and the pursuit of truth rule the day. The righteous indignation we feel when society members have been wronged knows no end to the wrath. We want to prevent the pain and suffering we've seen and felt up close. We identify with the pain, and perhaps we've experienced the same kind of pain ourselves. Perhaps it is our own desire to avoid future pain that drives us to expose, educate and improve our communities, and hopefully, even the world.

Despite a great deal of sadness and anger from covering some of the most depressing human and animal abuse stories on the planet, many reporters believe, like Anne Frank wrote in her diary, that people are basically good and want to do the right thing. Case studies in politics may seem like egomaniacs and narcissists rule the day. But hopefully, good prevails and the messengers are not killed in the process, either symbolically or in real life, as they sometimes are. In a world that grows more polarized, however, raging arguments develop a life of their own and facts can sometimes fall by the wayside in the passion of the moment. Faux news seeps onto our radar, and we may never be aware a story is false until way after the fact, the election or the event is well over with. If at all. The best protection is to follow the money and keep asking questions. Lots of questions.

People ask all the time, "How do you know anymore what is true and what is faux news?" The answer, as it always has been, is to get your facts from long-established, multiple, trusted and reliable sources. That's it.

Reporters are often controlled and ordered to do some stories with a certain focus, slant and agenda. But for the most part, at least for now, freedom of the press still rules in our culture. It is truth, justice and the American way, to quote Clark Kent from "Superman" that is at the driving power behind a reporter's desire to get at and fairly report the truth. Or so it was before Fox News invented the tagline after every radio news broadcast, "Fair and Balanced." I always thought that if a station or network had to say that, it probably wasn't. It was simply a way to quash the remote possibility and mounting criticisms that perhaps the news outlet wasn't doing as thorough reporting job as they should. Many reporters still feel as if they are called to the profession by God or divine intervention. It was and is our right as reporters to defend the First Amendment, to invade privacy, turn lives upside-down, bust in the doors, all in the pursuit of truth. It is about the checks and balances in our way of life that keeps our government and laws accountable and honest. In theory.

And so it goes with that pesky veganism. That concept that just won't go away. Veganism is the idea that humans don't need and should not exploit, use, wear or eat animals in any form or fashion. It is a lifestyle, not just a diet. It is the easiest thing you can do to improve your health, the planet and the lives of billions of animals slaughtered every year in and out of water, just for the latest fashions and our tastebuds. Not needed. Not necessary. Google "factory farming," and if those billions of images don't haunt your nightmares and make you go vegan immediately, I might buy you vegan dinners for a month. (I'm sure there will be a few holdouts.) But seriously. The more videos, photos, memes and images that are in your face, it is hard to stick your head in the sand and pretend not to see. You can't go back. I often say that the reason there are so many younger vegans than older is that they grew up in the YouTube generation. Once you've seen the images of baby chicks ground up on the first day of life because they serve no purpose for the egg industry since they'll never lay eggs, you can't ever erase it.

The motivation of this book, as might be obvious by now is somewhat, OK, completely selfish. I want the world oozing with more vegan men. It is really just this simple: I know how incredibly different and amazing it can be to have sex with a guy who can have a hard, pleasing erection and can keep it up. For a long time. I know how awful it is to have sex with a guy who can't. Ever.

We are often told erectile dysfunction is psychological and that it can be a self-perpetuating endless cycle. Perhaps. But perhaps I call B.S. most of the time.

Knowing what I know now, I suspect that every ex I had, if he'd known that cutting out the high-fat meats, chicken and pork, along with the eggs and cheese, would have greatly cleared out their arteries, reduced their cholesterol and improved blood flow, ED would have been a non-issue.

What does the canary in the coal mine mean for heart disease? Simply, it is the leading indicator of something big is about to happen. Little vessels get clogged and closed before those big ones do.

When my ex had his heart attack, during the 30 days I stayed with him in cardiac rehab, the director of the unit made rounds one night when my ex was in the room. She said to both of us not mincing words, "You've got to understand that husbands and significant others never listen to wives or partners. Never. So you need to listen to me. Change your diet. Your partner knows more about nutrition than almost anybody on our staff. Listen to her." Like his best friend who once said before the heart attack, "You live with one of the best vegan cookbook authors in America. Why don't you eat what she makes three times a day?" Suffice it to say, both comments went over like a lead balloon. But way, way before all that happened, as my ex and I discussed my growing vegan passion, he chuckled recalling that when he went to his various doctors to complain and eventually get treated for heart disease, that his failing penis may be the first clue that his heart was failing. When I tried to go there and help him, he wouldn't do it. He would even tell friends that he didn't have heart disease, even though he had been on the blood thinners, blood pressure meds, and cholesterol lowering drugs for decades since we first met. When I would confront him a time or two on that, he would simply say, "I haven't had a heart attack, so I don't have heart disease." What people do to deceive themselves, right?

Then there's the whole compassion, do unto others as you would have them do unto you, both in the human and non-human spectrum. To be blunt (get the idea you're going to get a lot of that in this book?) those vegans I know in the carnal and non-carnal way are gems of human beings. They are incredibly smart because they got to veganism on a primarily self-directed course. They swam up against the stream of conventional wisdom, and the strongly held beliefs of friends, family and their communities. Perhaps they woke up like Einstein one day and thought, it's just plain stupid not to be vegan because it is the smartest thing you can do, for animals, the planet and your health. But in the early days of veganism before there were studies on health and before we knew the earth was round, let alone in peril from human-caused animal agriculture run-off, people gave serious thought to the idea of the absurdity and pain caused by eating animals. In short, it was animal rights issues that prompted the early thinkers of the time to come to their own conclusions about why it made sense or didn't to eat animals and their fluids. They walked a mile in the animal's shoes or to put in animal terms, hooves.

The vegan men of today who arrived at the table through their own reading, watching movies, videos and involvement in their own vegan communities are to be celebrated and held up as role models. Some men have become vegan because of their woman. Some did it all on their own. And vice versa. Since more women are vegan than men, these men who did it on their own, or simultaneously with their partner, are few and far between. Even if they got to veganism with the assistance of a significant other in their life, their ability to go there and stay there is to be appreciated no matter how and why it happened.

As a result, at least in my experience and those women I know, men committed to veganism are in short supply and in hot demand. The consequence is that many vegan men rather enjoy their local celebrityness and the resulting lines out their front doors. They are compassionate and giving in all aspects of their lives, from volunteering at their local vegfest, farm sanctuaries, taking in strays, building cat shelters, and taking on leadership roles on their local animal rights or vegan lifestyle boards. They'll plan meetups and do some of the heavy lifting it takes to organize community events. There's not a mean bone in their body. They are often fabulous chefs because they've read the same books their partners have read. Or at least they've watched their partners cook very carefully, or helped with the prep. Some even do all the clean-up uttering that wonderful phrase, "It's the least I can do." You have a friend for life and a keeper if your meal recipient helps you scratch clean-up detail off your list.

When it comes down to it, these activists are prepared and often do, dig deep into their pockets, if they have the means to support some of the many vegan causes and especially sanctuaries. The most appealing men and women truly put their money where their mouths are and often create, organize and run sanctuaries. There's nothing sexier or harder than a sweaty guy or gal who devotes their life, day after to day, to the grueling regimen of maintaining a sanctuary. They are also doing the hardest work on the planet. Whether they have much energy at the end of the day after such a rigorous routine may be subject of debate. But of course, with a balanced and healthy vegan diet, hopefully energy for sex is not an issue much of the time for even these heavy lifters.

To a vegan woman, there's nothing more appealing than a thoughtful, compassionate man who can prepare a delicious vegan dinner all on his own. The flip side I've seen is that some guys who may not have enjoyed such notoriety and a huge selection of women to choose from in their ancient past, get a little overwhelmed. Sometimes this can go to their head, making it swell or just messing it up a bit. Scoundrel is a word I've heard to describe the classic vegan prince who has so many ladies to choose from and just can't or chooses not to quite pick one. Or several. If you are involved with such a guy, you may want to check yourself regularly for STDs. Humor aside, I'm probably not telling you anything you don't already know. A guy who has it all in the vegan universe–he's come there on his own journey and is knowledgeable and consistent with his vegan values is irresistible for many vegan women. A guy you don't have to teach? Beyond cool. No wonder he is sought after.

To a vegan man, having a meal, especially a hot meal prepared 1-3 times a day, or even a week, is Nirvana. While this is really old school, it is true that the way to anyone's heart is through their stomachs. Spoiler alert: It works in reverse for women, too. For busy men or women, any kind of help is welcome. If you enjoy cooking, sharing your love and enthusiasm in the kitchen is golden. Don't hesitate to build your partner's confidence, however. Especially if he or she is a little lacking in experience cooking, assigning simple tasks like mincing onions or garlic can go a long way toward building a partnership of cooperation, skill sets and lifelong learning. The vegan experience goes way beyond the kitchen. But not everyone understands when they begin with those first baby-steps, that we all took baby-steps at the beginning of our journeys.

I remember after teaching cooking classes for years and being on a date with a poor guy who really wanted to learn about veganism but didn't understand why it wasn't cool to send a vegan woman a photo of a donkey who was forced to provide rides to parade participants on a hot, Florida, 4th of July 6-mile route. How do you teach that kind of compassion? Either you're born with it or you get up to speed pretty quickly when you transition. So many videos exist now on YouTube and all over social media it doesn't take long to get educated quickly. However, in the more mature age groups, computer skills and access to social media vary widely. The frustration for some women may be as much about their partners not being computer savvy enough to be able to access and watch and learn from all the incredible resources we now have. With smart phones, we have such access. Videos and movies that could not have been attempted 20 or even 10 years ago document with pinpoint accuracy what happens to animals in all kinds of conditions.

Some men get interested in veganism because their partner has brought them along kicking and screaming. If the relationship fails, often veganism fails for the man as well. Sometimes he was just trying to do "it" to please his lady. As with so many things, you have to please yourself first. You can't get off any addiction, alcohol, smoking or meat and dairy because you want to please another. Having a partner you want to please may help and be part of motivation and inspiration to go vegan. But it can never be the sole reason. The decision to go and more importantly, remain vegan in the long term, must come from deep within. The long term decision and commitment depends on how much the partner gets the message and is committed to the cause for all the right reasons, however he or she defines it. One study even shows that those who choose veganism for ethics rather than health tend to be long term vegans more so than those who go there for only for health reasons. However, in my experience in teaching cooking classes, I knew many people who remained vegan for the long term based on their near-death experiences. As I was fond of saying, people get desperate on their death beds. It can definitely work both ways. One woman who was given up for dead in my Physicians Committee for Responsible Medicine's Cancer Project cooking class had been diagnosed with multiple myeloma, one of the more fatal forms of bone cancer. After 8 months, she lost 120 pounds she needed to lose, loved the food and never counted calories. 13 years later, she is still alive and well, and says that she is still "a raving vegan." Results are typical. Ask your doc if plants are right for you.

One of the more interesting things that happens is that men who maybe are going along with the whole vegan "thang" changing their diet for their woman, find themselves weeks or months later in a situation at a restaurant or public gathering where they dig right into that pizza or steak they really thought they were missing. The reaction on their faces when they experience stomach discomfort is memorable. That "aha" moment when they say, "Ya know, I really don't like the taste of meat anymore." Hopefully they will get the "vegan for animals" connection soon. But if they at least remain on the diet, one more vegan in the world is always a good thing, no matter the reason. We all get to vote with our wallets three or more times a day. And that's where it really counts. When demand for plant foods increases, this is what truly creates an impact and change. The supply of animal products decreases, and the farmers who created that supply, will change what they do for a living, converting to plant production. We are already seeing this happening big time as headlines are oozing with farmers who are freeing cows from their imprisonment, turning their land into sanctuaries and "raising" alternative milks by planting almonds, seeds and other plants that can easily provide milk. Rowdy Girl Sanctuary is one example of a very publicized cattle ranch turned plant farm by a gutsy wife who said she couldn't take it anymore, and much to everyone's surprise, her husband listened and changed his ways, big time.

However, we do need more men who take the ball (and their balls) and run with it. I'm hoping that if meat-eating men realize that their erectile dysfunction can be cured so simply in just a few meals, that will result in a line out the door of beautiful inside and out women who want to share that journey. That is one sure-fire way we'll end up with more vegan men. It's so ridiculously simple. No more meds. And a crop of healthy, smart women begging you for a date. What could be better? When was the last time you heard a doctor say, "Go on a vegan diet and call me in the morning?" No money in broccoli.

What is sexy is defined differently for all of us. But in a changing, hurting world, veganism answers so many problems and is the answer to many of our world's ills. To cause no harm to ourselves and others is a powerful place to live our lives. To support the work of those who devote their working and/ or volunteer lives to saving animals, the planet and our health is a real turn-on and a great opportunity if you are so lucky to live around such dedicated souls.

A word about sexual designations. For the sake of simplicity, I write from my own experience of being female and dealing with men in heterosexual relationships. That has been my lifelong orientation. But the genders as I refer to them here can be reversed, interchanged or be the same. However it works best in your situation and orientation. All good.

I have never had or wanted to have sex with a woman. So I can't really compare the experience of one woman to another except in the interviews I have done. Because I have experienced different men, vegan and not, I can offer my observations of the differences from my perspective. As a result, what I write about here reflects my first-hand account of the very obvious differences among men and their adoption of a vegan diet. All in the name of research and reporting, of course. Different women want and desire different things in their relationships. While I suspect my experiences are not uncommon, I can only write from the center of the hurricane of whirling observations and admitted bias toward what has worked and hasn't worked for me over decades of sometimes very painful losses and realizations.

I developed a survey that I gave to a number of people who contributed their ideas to this book. I wanted very much to address some of the main issues facing the LGBT community. But I was unable to find anyone willing to answer the survey questions or contribute to the text. Maybe in the sequel.

With the hindsight of 20/20 vision, I highly recommend that if you are vegan, do your best to find a vegan partner, or one who is very, very vegan friendly, loves to go to vegan restaurants and will eat vegan at home most, if not all of the time. At the very least, he or she should take you to a vegan restaurant or make you a fab vegan dinner on your birthday. We are a growing world community now, and with some of the resources provided in this book and online, you can find your vegan soulmate, life partner, significant other, or local and distant communities to make the journey less lonely, more fun and rewarding.

CHAPTER 2

Invading Privacy to Tell the Truth

The first reason why vegans do it better is because they are generally, though not always, in better physical shape. Studies show their hearts are more fully functional and they have lower body weights than non-vegans. This generally allows them to participate in sports or fitness activities that will help keep them in better and even great physical shape. The stamina that allows them to be in great shape out of bed transfers immediately into the bedroom. If you have ever had sex with a long-time smoker who has beginning emphysema, you know exactly what I'm talking about. It is difficult for them to breathe and in some cases, impossible to reach an orgasm because they can't breathe deeply enough to get there.

Although I haven't seen studies, there is anecdotal evidence that vegans who smoke can still have amazing sex with erections lasting an hour or longer. You heard me right. Vegans and animal activists who smoke. Conventional wisdom dictates that if you eat a vegan diet which is presumably healthy, then how could you possibly smoke since smoking has been linked to almost every disease under the sun, especially cancer? If you Google animal testing by cigarette companies, there are ample links to evidence that cigarette companies do some of the worst testing on animals. Unfortunately, we lived in a time when cigarette companies were allowed to pass out free cigarettes to high school kids at dance clubs. Nicotine addiction is one of the toughest addictions to break. In older generations, cigarettes were easy to get, become addicted to, and poison control directors were not running around with cancer-riddled lungs preserved in a baggie filled with formaldehyde, as they do now to scare children away from smoking. In spite of overwhelming evidence of cigarette companies testing on animals, a few of the most vocal, staunchest vegans can't or won't kick the habit.

The biggest obstacle to some people switching to a vegan diet is that they live in fear that they will develop a severe protein deficiency from not eating enough animal protein. If you ask most vegans what question they get the most, it is almost always the "where do you get your protein" question. We all have our 10-second retorts. This is the most commonly used answer: The largest, studliest animals on the planet are plant-eaters. They're vegan. They're beautiful. Think of an elephant, a rhinoceros, giraffe, hippopotamus, wildebeest, bison, horse, manatee, yak, deer and some whales. All plant eaters. Some are aggressive, some are dangerous, all are magnificent, powerful and definitely not lacking in protein or energy.

They have no protein deficiencies and have plenty of energy to run, jump, leap, reach, and procreate and breastfeed their young. Or another popular retort is, "I get my protein where your protein gets their protein." All plant foods have protein. A tiny banana has a gram of it. Vegans get enough protein. Plenty of protein. Even the mainstream, bought-off, in-bed-with-politicians USDA says Americans are too obsessed and get too much protein. There's some real confirmation, if you ever needed it.

The next step--endurance and stamina.

To watch TV commercials in the US, you would think having children would be a miracle short of immaculate conceptions the way nobody can reportedly get it up. Western culture has been inundated with erectile dysfunction commercials that promote "staying power" for those whose blood flow doesn't quite make it all over their body to the most important organs for optimal sexual function. Certainly the emotional component gives staying power to the physical parts of our bodies. Running memes suggest that intensely physical sport is very much a mind over matter battle. Any endurance sport can sport the same argument.

To a point. With sex, it may be more about blood getting and staying in our appendages. In fact, here comes that refrain again: it's all about blood flow. After all, the muscles in the penis respond by expanding and becoming erect as blood flows into the penis--as much 8 times more than what's there under flaccid conditions. With such a huge network in the penis, clogged arteries may create a work stoppage, or a downright strike.

One of the stars of the vegan lecture circuit, Dr. Terry Mason, the Chief Operator Officer for the Chicago Department of Public Health, has also been a urological surgeon for 30 years. He runs around the country showing incredibly graphic videos of penile implant surgeries. He concludes that presentation, which, trust me, will never leave your brain with, "All men ought to be required to watch this. If they knew what was in store as a result of eating an artery-clogging diet, they would change their diet to plant-based in a heartbeat!"

Dr. Mason's work and talk is clearly an indication that most men have no idea that eating a diet filled with animal products clogs arteries and vessels everywhere. The shortage of vegan men may be in part, responsible for the lack of knowledge and experience among populations as a whole. While opinions vary depending what link and study you view, it does seem to be that there are more vegan women than men as we age, and more women than men in general. Women are still outliving the guys. The gender gap has been widely studied, and in almost every city in the US, there are far more women than men--as many as 29% more women than men with McAllen, Texas, topping that list. If you're a woman and really want to get depressed, you can search a census page called "Where the Boys Are" and find the number of single women to every 100 single men in your state or county. The odds are really depressing in Florida. Sarasota County leads that list with 70 men to every 100 women. As for vegan ratios, depending what study or article you're looking at, it is estimated that between 70-80% of all vegans in the US are women. At many events I attend and observe, this statistic seems to hold.

There is a huge movement afoot to recruit more vegan men. I heard this overtly expressed first years ago by Amanda Smith, who organizes "Get Healthy Marshall TX" and their incredible fun-filled vegan weekend, "Healthfest." Others have also said that we need to recruit more vegan men. The ratio of men to women decreases even more as we age. My goal, as I suspect yours is if you are vegan, is to convert as many vegans as possible in as short a time as possible. We understand the urgency for our health and the environment. By going vegan, as studies, experts and even the United Nations said in a report way back in 2010, we can reduce the impact of climate change, rainforest destruction, and pollution, while saving water and other resources. Exploiting animals for food produces more greenhouse gas emissions than all of the cars, planes, and other forms of transportation combined.

As rights get stripped and agencies and programs defunded, the urgency screams even louder for the sake of animals, the environment and our health. If you are not vegan, but at least vegan curious, perhaps this book's title piqued your interest for yet one more reason that a vegan diet and lifestyle might work for you.

Bottom line, if more men truly believed they could last longer, sustain an erection, a firm, hard erection, and the other delights of sex without the crappy drugs with their dire 4-hour warnings that are as common as water in our culture, the line to veganism would be endless. ED drug companies would shut down, and maybe, just maybe, some pharmaceutical companies which depend hugely on ED drugs as their main income stream, would declare bankruptcy.

In case you're unfamiliar with ED drugs, or haven't heard the blaring of their TV commercials over the decades, many of them come with a final warning, "If you have an erection lasting more than 4 hours, call your doctor." Or as some of my vegan women friends now say, "Call me."

I'm guessing longer, harder erections could be a huge enticement in ways that nobody has ever written about before. Recent studies show that millennials, those who were born roughly between 1980 and 2004, aren't really interested in sex, especially not as much as generations before them. Is it because they are oversaturated, and have been overloaded from an early age with sex in the media, making it overrated? Is it the plethora of ED commercials that made them think that if sex is going to fail under "natural" conditions, as they know it, i.e. on a meat and dairy-based diet, what's the point? If you have to take meds to make "it" work, why bother? "It" is harder...or not? Forgive the pun.

Are millennials truly less interested in sex than their parents? Hard to believe, with the way ads everywhere put it out there. Is it that they just have no idea what they're missing because they've never had it, or had it very great? Is it so available that familiarity breeds contempt? These are not simple questions with easy answers. Just putting it out there gives us all food for thought.

Pundits give all kinds of possible reasons from kids have nothing to prove, or that they just prefer to work at a career instead of a relationship since they're less interested in marriage. There are many studies, reports and articles showing that the more we are connected online, the less we are connected in real life. How often does it happen that teens sitting right next to one another text to communicate? As one millennial I coached in high school track confided during a long run, known for its power on the brain to release inhibitions to talk, much like alcohol, she said, "Our generation just doesn't know how to talk to each other." Another consideration is that when teens prefer to text than talk, it allows them a way to hide from each other. Texting allows for total control of their message, whereas an old fashioned phone call, or in-person chat might be a little more scary and revealing, given that both or multiple people vie for control of the conversation. What this means is younger generations are losing their ability to look into their partner's eyes and talk directly to them. They have isolated themselves completely from even the ones they love. Being "out of touch" grows in meaning.

Another obstacle that makes at least the consequences of having sex not so fun is considering what kind a world will be around in 20, 40 or 60 years when today's pregnant couples are grandparents. Frankly, looking at the future of the planet, between the predicted environmental degradation, world strife and seemingly unstoppable conflict, many are asking with more realism than generations before them, "Who would want to bring children into such a world that could very well die in doomsday predictions." Facebook and Twitter, which often link to graphic videos on YouTube are great educational tools, but they also zero in on the stark reality of the future that lies ahead for humans, non-human animals and the planet. These are questions and issues I can't answer. Only you, can dig deep to figure these solutions out.

Not Tonight Dear, Or Ever Again

Back to the matter at hand. One can also wonder, if the parts worked better, more efficiently, or if there were more rewards in terms of sexual gratification, would sexual partners be more interested or interesting? Would a great sexual relationship be worth the investment of time? If the nest was deeply satisfying at home, would there be a need to fly or even look elsewhere?

Despite the male brain being hardwired to look at women every which way including sideways, I say yes. As my sexual partners declined in ability and then in interest, the excuses and rationalizations from both of us set in. "Not tonight dear, I have a headache," turned into, "It's OK. Whatever you do or not, is fine with me. No judgement zone here." And finally, "You know, what matters is emotional intimacy, friendship and compatibility. Sex is greatly overrated anyway."

"Snore rooms" have become a thing. An empty nester's child's bedroom was converted as a safe haven from an incessantly and loudly snoring partner, usually the man, but not always. Articles in home decorating magazines exploded about the joy a woman felt as she redecorated a snoring room for just herself. Wonderful.

Why do people snore? When you Google that question, you get a sanitized answer like this, "snoring is caused by a partially closed upper airway (the nose and throat). Everyone's neck muscles relax during sleep, but sometimes they relax so much that the upper airway partly closes and becomes too narrow for enough air to travel through to the lungs."

Other risk factors include alcohol consumption, allergies, nasal obstruction, muscle relaxants and smoking. But the biggest factor in snoring is obesity. Excess fat doesn't just land on the belly and other common sites. It can build in extra fat layers on the inside of the throat causing constriction.

Is it part of the aging process? A little perhaps. But I would argue that it really is not. While yes, you often hear the argument that everyone is different, I have been so astounded in my observations, that I can't believe the age of my vegan partners. They have been, as many vegans are, slim and at a healthy weight. They had no excess fat in their throats and were quiet as a lamb when it came to snoring. I'm guessing they had no excess fat clogging arteries, veins and other vessels to interfere with sexual performance. Yes, that's how good it was.

How bad was it? While this is not a blanket statement, non-vegans tend to snore more. In my experience, snoring seemed to also correlate with ED. Sexual performance was so rare in my last few decades of life, it was often nonexistent. It was so rare, with all that ED that I frequently found myself feeling with non-vegan partners, based on performance alone, I couldn't believe I ever had children. Semen with child-producing sperm can still be ejected from a lackluster penis. Perhaps with a struggling penis, it seems that the odds are against being fruitful and multiplying. An uphill battle of sorts.

In some cases, when a man experiences repeated ED problems, he uses the excuse to move to another bedroom to avoid another failure and perpetuating the cycle. If this becomes chronic, sex falls off the radar completely.

In the words of one converted vegan who is now a believer, he advises: Women: If you want to help keep your guy feeling good about himself and his sexual prowess, encourage him change his diet.

The Fountain of Youth

A healthful, balanced vegan diet, rich with antioxidants and phytochemicals is well-known for increasing vitality on the inside and outside. Vegans often look younger than their years. So many people refuse to believe my chronological age based on looks alone. After competing in the National Senior Games and placing 7th in my age group in the 1500 meters, 10th in the 400, I received a survey as did all participants. We had to answer questions on a survey about our health and fitness, including things like our resting heart rate. Based on my answers, I received results back that said, "Your chronological age is 62, but you have the fitness of an average 26 year-old." Point being, nobody is measuring my sexual prowess. However, I've had more than one partner comment that my flexibility, stamina and endurance in bed are probably "because of your running. And diet." It has to work with others who are equally fit. But even for the casual or occasional vegan weekend athlete or exerciser, the results of a clean diet pay off without all the kinds of workouts and racing I do. One of my matches in a dating service said the reason he was so interested in me, aside from the fact that I was the healthiest and trimmest of anyone he had dated in in a year, was that I was interesting and could bike 6-10 miles a day with him. He said that no one else came close in comparing in energy and enthusiasm for life.

What makes me different from a doctor or cardiologist who is focused on the research, peer-reviewed science and clinical studies is that sadly, I have lived in real life, the experience of both vegan and non-vegan men. The biggest obstacle in writing this story is how I tell that tale and maintain and protect privacy. Sharing details of my personal life is not something I've ever wanted to do. As a member of a family that led a public life in politics in the Midwest, and then myself as a TV reporter for 18 years, we fought to keep details of our personal lives as best we could, out of the public eye. With the development of computers, that became increasingly hard to do. Social media became a job prerequisite, and before long, it seemed that nothing was private. "Your followers and fans want to know intimate details of your life," experts advised. Really? Must I? And indeed, when I tried to get my first book published, it was turned down for a year, because all the publishers cared about was how many friends I had on Facebook, and how many tweets a day I tweeted. I paid someone to take me beyond the social media skills of snooping on my children to make sure they were OK. As the admin of more than a dozen Facebook pages now, I sometimes wonder what I got myself into. But it is a necessary of evil of being an author. It is also the single best way to spread the vegan message and health benefits.

I advised and did media consulting and training for Physicians Committee for Responsible Medicine, one of the country's oldest and super effective animal rights and vegan health non-profits. After leaving mainstream reporting in the dust, I was privileged to train some of the most prolific and vocal plant-based doctors who bucked conventional medicine, the pharmaceutical industry and their mainstream pharma-paid-for medical training, and did what was right for their patients. I had heard PCRM's president, Dr. Neal Barnard speak in my hometown, St. Louis, in the 1980's. His messages of animal protection and linking a vegan diet to optimal health resonated as I watched so many in my family get really sick or really dead.

After I left TV, I spent 5 years as a financial consultant at Smith Barney where I focused on helping clients invest in socially responsible companies that did great things for the environment while avoiding tobacco and alcohol (the legal definition of SRI), and for those clients who wanted it, companies that tested on animals. Companies like Proctor and Gamble were out. When I went to St. Louis Animal Rights Team meetings in the 1980's where I first heard Dr. Barnard, they passed out magnets and pins that said "Died." Designed to look like P & G's popular product "Tide," it was easy for me to connect the dots and understand why so many clients demanded that their investment portfolios remain "mission consistent" with their values. In that horrific investment year, 2001, I was the number one market performer in my branch. All I got for that honor was an email to prove it. Investment firms weren't necessarily crazy that the public know that their highest earning financial consultants weren't necessarily the highest performers when it came to how well they did for their clients' portfolios.

I eventually became convinced that how well I did for clients was inversely correlated to how well I did for myself. After never earning more than $20,000 in my 5-year stint there, I called it quits and began doing media consulting full-time. My first day "on the job," I emailed Dr. Barnard and said, "I know you are completely, wonderfully eloquent and don't need my services, but if anyone on your staff could benefit from my years in TV, what makes a good story and how to appear relaxed while getting your message across in 10 seconds or less, I'd be happy to help." Within weeks, I was on a plane for what would become several sessions over the next few years of media training I did for PCRM staff and health care professionals who wanted more experience with the media. After my years in the media, I knew as much as anyone about how much newsmakers need to share in order to capture the public interest. That's why I began brainstorming about all the different myths I could begin to bust by defining activism on a whole new level. I asked myself, as I would encourage you to do, "What I can I do best to advance this cause of veganism? How can I best use my abilities, skills and talents? I do believe that protesting can be effective, but showing up at a 5K race with 300 to 3000 people on any given Florida weekend, wearing a neon vegan shirt with "Eat Vegan on $4 a Day" on it was my passion. The message got double-takes and if I don't have at least 3 people come up to me on race day, stare at my shirt and go, "How?" I feel my mission has not been accomplished.

The feedback I often get, especially as I age, is that I am a walking, sometimes running, talking billboard and poster child for the many physical and health benefits eating and living a vegan lifestyle can bring over decades.

While protecting my privacy and those who have been the source of some of the information for this book, I also recognize I need to spill the beans on the most important details that can help others recognize that misery is not inevitable. You can have a fabulous life, and a great sex life if you are willing to be open to the ideas and concepts here. I think that the worst thing I ever saw in my non-vegan sex life was one partner who asked me to help him administer a shot of viagra into his penis. I've had a lot of strange requests in my life. But I couldn't do it. For a lot of reasons. Mainly, knowing what he had eaten all his life, and how he continued to eat, his condition was preventable. Call me heartless and lacking in compassion. I couldn't go to that table. But there's a high likelihood that "supplementation" is what's ahead if you or your partner isn't vegan. Not my idea of a good time, and I'm guessing, not yours either.

To the extent that dirty and clean laundry is aired, it is the price paid to get more individuals, couples and families happier, satisfied and positively focused. Saving a few animals and the planet along the way, is a small price to pay. I hope my ex-husbands and significant and insignificant others agree.

Attitude is Altitude

Just because you eat a vegan diet doesn't mean it is a healthy vegan diet. Just because you're vegan, doesn't mean you'll always have stellar sex. Just because you have picked a vegan partner doesn't guarantee wedded or unwedded bliss. Because I'm writing what I know, I sadly admit that I know this topic better than I want to. Way better than any topic I've written about so far. Again, sadly. Why sadly, one of my editors asked? I had parents who celebrated 64 years of mostly wedded bliss before my mom left this world first. They had public displays of affection until their dying days. Dad fondly spoke about her "swivel hips" and other attributes on most days. Those of us who had such role models probably hold on to some fantasy that life can be like that--happy with one soulmate for a lifetime. But for most of us, 64 years is not going to happen.

Dealing with ED whether it was the cause or the symptom of unhappy times and deep-seated negative emotions, derails too many relationships that perhaps, might have stood a longer test of time. "Serial monogamy" is the term created to describe a lifetime of relationship bouncing. The extent to which social monogamy is observed in animals varies across all animal species. Interestingly, more than 90 percent of bird species are socially monogamous, compared to only 3 percent of mammalian species and up to 15 percent of primate species. Research is mixed on when humans developed monogamy for a lifetime, or a long time. However we process or define it for ourselves, having a romantic dream of how blissful pairing plays out in our lifetime is a cross between a Disney fantasy and reality TV drama. No matter how we justify that it is part of our species' behavior, breakups are painful and not how the script was supposed to play out.

The scariest part of writing this story is revealing how I know what I know. But once the truth hit me in the face, I became so angry there was no choice but to write the truth. Busting vegan myths. That's what needs to be done. Simply, here's how it went.

Let's just say, I've been married several times and had numerous relationships, as many people do by the time they mature. As one of my daughters says, "Well, Mom, at least that means you've been loved that many times. Some people never know love." Great. I guess. OK. I'll take that to the bank as I try to focus on the positive. However, I must admit, when filling out those online dating questionnaires and struggling to be honest, but maybe not too honest about what I am really searching for, the answer is clear after all these years: A kind, giving, self-educated vegan who knows how to cook, respects and loves me for who I am, faults and all. It would have been nice to have lived with that person for 50 or 60 years, like my parents before me. I didn't even know what the word vegan meant in my twenties. Most of us didn't. But I would have accepted someone who at least had the capacity to grow into it, as many of us have.

At this point in life, marriage isn't even on the radar. But I believe that partnerships, especially with vegans, can be exhilarating and beneficial to both partners in so many ways when living alone is, frankly, lonely. It just is. I can't tell you how many married men and women have said things like, "Oh, just don't focus so much on the end result. Don't worry about marriage or even being in a relationship." My retort, "Easy for you to say, you're married. Or in a relationship." Nobody disagrees with me at that point.

For a while, I lived in a beautiful microscopic one-bedroom condo on the Gulf of Mexico.

The complex had an abundance of about 20 single women, and 2 bachelors. One of them, drove up as I moved in and offered to help me unload. He'd had prostate cancer and heard in his hospital recovery class that a vegan diet was effective for preventing recurrences of cancer. He had heard that I had been a trained cooking instructor for PCRM's The Cancer Project, and that I was a runner. On move-in day, when I pulled up in my "veganmobile" with all my vegan magnets on the car, he was ready to help me unload my life's possessions. As an avid biker wanting to maintain his health, he was only too eager to pump me for information and prepare vegan meals.

But he was also very sought after sexually and otherwise, not only locally, but in his hometown as well, where he returned 6 months out of the year. I was warned that he was a nice guy, but I would be the flavor of the month, and that his condo was a revolving door. Totally true.

In my searching for places to live after I was divorced, I went to one new complex and the saleswoman said, "Oh, you'll love it here. There are so many single women." "What about men?" I quipped. "We're working on that," she responded and changed the topic. Then sometime in the following year, I was not surprised to read a story that the nearest largest city to my condo had one of the highest ratios of women to men: 130 women to every man. Facebook lit up that day with men promising to move here. I have stopped holding my breath, however.

In each of my marriages and the few relationships I had before I got married and in-between, erectile dysfunction was always part of the equation. It was almost as if it was part of the "aging process." But at 28? How did we become so callous and disconnected from our bodies that ED and the plague of commercials on television became the new normal? And that we accepted this routine diagnosis as a standard part of life in our twenties. ED drugs hadn't been invented yet. But we somehow were told we had to live with it. Outrageous!

Personally, the only exception to my erectile dysfunction business-as-usual lifestyle was a guy who ate mostly vegan, though I never put two and two together. But I, like most American and Western women accepted ED as a way of life. Gone were the virile men of our teens (if you had sex that early, which I did not), twenties and if you're lucky, thirties. By 40, as the birthday party favors of the time said, you were "over the hill." Geriatric sex became a term jokingly, but frequently used to describe the half-hearted attempts to have sex in an aging population addicted to meat and dairy. Except that only I, and some of my vegetarian and vegan friends were just beginning to explore those connections. As ED took over our lives, we knew nothing of these magical pills that could "reverse" the limp attempts that were the accepted way of American life.

Home porn was part of the scene too, as our men lived vicariously through the twenty-something writhing, flailing bodies on screen, perfectly positioning themselves in every way possible. And they expected and demanded wives to watch under the guise of, "It'll help you too." Sex was mainly a spectator sport interspersed between Monday night football and rowdy hockey games. Go Blues! Go Rams! Ramming porn down my throat was not going to happen on our scrimmage line, though.

Then it happened. My ex grew increasingly intolerant and impatient with my including animal rights into my vegan-for-health talks. My books were debunking vegan myths--the misconception that a vegan diet was expensive, or that you couldn't live with others who didn't eat vegan, or that the Paleo fad was something new, when it was nothing more than Atkins or the Zone diet a little cleaned up, repackaged and remarketed all over again. Even though his friends and healthcare professionals told him that to avoid continued heart disease and another heart attack, he ought go easy or give up animal consumption in favor of plants, at some point, it no longer mattered. But even before the heart attack, his support of my activities waned. Not once did he ever suggest going to a vegan restaurant, and when I suggested it, he nixed it. I should have left in those moments.

But once in a committed relationship, especially marriage, which is not so easy to toss aside, I kept hoping. And hoping. As in so many relationships, women often think we can fix it, if we make the right meal, do the right thing and keep smiling.

Running for Fitness and Sexuality

I really hated running as a kid, but when I moved to Florida, the year-round great weather allowed me to start training more. Running burned calories at twice the speed of walking. So once I forced myself to do it, found some good music to distract me from the perceived boredom, I fell into an almost daily running pattern. I battled weight big time as child and yo-yo dieted as was typical for children of the 60's who survived happily on all 28 flavors of Baskin Robbins. As was also typical for the times, when I went whining to my doctor about my weight, he prescribed amphetamines which worked wonders suppressing appetite for a couple of weeks, but once the meds ended, appetites came screaming back, as did any lost weight, and then some.

When I finally got my weight under control through diet and a healthy running schedule, I eventually went to races and started placing in my age group, much to my surprise. I never could have placed when I was a young meat-eater. Because there was less competition in the older age groups, I started placing in races and then began wearing vegan shirts to races. I would joke that winning or placing in my age group was simply just about showing up. That always gets a laugh when I say that. But it really isn't true.

At my 11th half marathon, a popular jaunt in Sarasota, 33 other women finished ahead of me. But here's how I rationalize that. 1) I hadn't trained at all running around the country on book tour and constantly on social media for myself and my publisher, 2) The longest distance I'd put in before the 13.1 miles was a 10K, or 6.2 miles. I did that the week before the half marathon, which is not great training theory, since I should have been tapering. In theory, best running practice is to clock a 10 mile run before trying to do 13+. Oh well. I was busy writing this and other books. The week after the half marathon, despite my personal trainer saying, "You're not planning to race next weekend, are you?" I did, and got first in my age group at another 10K. Because I travel so much, I rationalized, I have to get my running and racing in when I can.

The few vegans I've met at races have all been women with only one exception. Sometimes they'll tap me on the shoulder from behind as I'm running and gesture, "Me too!" Or they'll see my bright vegan shirt after the race and strike up a conversation. While I've been lucky to run at some plant-based 5Ks nationally and have met a few well-known male vegan runners such as Gene Baur, president of Farm Sanctuary and running legends Rich Roll and Brendan Brazier, I have never had a male vegan runner tap me on the shoulder at a race and say "Me too!" In one instance, a guy who had lost a great deal of weight going plant based shared his story with me after a race when he saw my vegan shirt.

My vegan running shirts with their loud slogans and pictures, have spurred so many questions and conversations at races. I realized that my running was becoming my activism. I would be standing around after placing in my age group at a race, one of the 115 or more times I had done that since 2006 "just" on plants, and someone would invariably come up to me, as I'm holding the award medal in my hand, stare at my "Eat Vegan on $4 a Day" bright yellow neon shirt and say, "You can't run or race on a vegan diet." I would use the opportunity to engage and educate. My mission was born. I realized how many people believed so many myths about veganism. Running seemed to be the fastest way to dispel the weakling who doesn't get enough protein myth. At every talk I gave, I began to flex my biceps and say as they popped up, "Does it look like I have a protein deficiency? Do you know anyone who has been diagnosed with a protein deficiency? (Rarely would someone raise their hand. I always wondered if it was really true.) Do you know anyone who has been diagnosed with cancer, heart disease and diabetes? That's where we should be focusing our stress and nervous, worrying energy."

Losing a Marriage to Veganism

As one of my marriages crumbled, the thought of donating my relationship to my growing passion certainly crossed my mind. Did my "cult" claim our marriage, as he would accuse. Did I lose my marriage to veganism, I wondered in my darker moments. My family of origin's "black sheep" label came roaring back with a vengeance. How many of you have been adorned with one or both of those labels? But of course, it is never that simple.

My ex initially came to some of my early races. Although I never did, he grew weary of the same questions that came my way and my same answers. More importantly, as my health and athleticism continued to maintain and improve, and his declined and devolved into a heart attack with fat-clogged arteries screaming for bypasses, his resentment was seething below the surface, and then blatantly obvious when people like his friend asked him point blank why he just didn't eat what I made. When confronted, he would blame his bad treatment of me on his mother and ex-wife. In joint therapy, he would be reminded constantly through many examples of our reality that he brought up that I was neither of those two awful women his past life, and a pretty nice, thoughtful gal in his current life perfectly willing to fix him 3 healthy meals a day. In fact, I was always happy to fix his meals, if they were vegan. In our divided household, I would fix his vegan side dishes which tended to be mostly grits and a whole grain, if I could sneak in something other than grits swimming in dairy butter. Yes, there were times when I would prepare fish when he refused to eat anything vegan, which was most of the time. After he had his heart attack, one of the doctors asked when he last ate something green, as in a vegetable. He laughed and said he couldn't remember.

In short, my thriving on a vegan lifestyle was a threat and constant reminder of how his own lifelong choices had failed him. Growing up as a Florida native, fishing from early childhood, even as an educated college graduate who had a great career that could have easily left him open to learning and experiencing at least the health benefits of a vegan lifestyle, change was never a serious option.

How we get into toxic relationships is the subject of many books. Being vegan, or even being in a relationship with another vegan does not guarantee a lifetime of bliss. But as we age, hope springs eternal that we can somehow repair or fix the fissures of failure. Or we rationalize, maybe we can just put up with it as long as the positives still outweigh the negatives. Or sometimes we just stay stuck in a relationship thinking, it won't be any different with anyone else. Or perhaps we just run out of energy believing that it's easier to stay home with the unconditional fur ball animal love on the couch. If a person doesn't get the vegan thing, or show any interest in learning, the hardest decision you may have to make is cutting the cord and going it alone. So much easier said than done. I know.

Beyond Circus Protesting

While I had protested the abuse of animals, especially elephants in circuses, with my babes in arms decades ago, my ex conveniently forgot that those experiences and feelings had very much been a part of my background and education as I became more outspoken on the lecture circuit. I was doing nothing more than connecting dots between animal rights, health and the environment, as many of us do. Indeed, going vegan solves everything, if you think about it. As the most respected scientists and studies, including the United Nations have said, going vegan does more to reduce our carbon footprint. Those who grew up in the YouTube generation see the many kinds of atrocities that are recorded with smart phones. It's hard to watch continued animal abuse. It is hard to ever forget the wailing sound a mama cow has as her baby is ripped from her breast on the first day of life so that her milk can be taken away and given to humans instead of her own baby. As a long-time leader of the breastfeeding organization, La Leche League, the idea of any mammalian baby being ripped from its mother anytime, is so disgusting and repulsive. The Facebook group, "Mothers Against Dairy," is but one large outcry of the same feelings any mother must have, regardless of the species and whether she breastfed or not.

As a former television investigative reporter who took days to design a purse that an undercover video camera would fit in, I was in awe of how well a smart phone camera could record atrocities we knew were happening, but couldn't record because the technology wasn't there yet. I covered some of the worst animal abuse stories of my time when I was a television reporter. We got more calls than any other story I'd ever done when we showed partially disintegrated, charred dogs and cats being improperly disposed at the city dump. Of course, the stories back in those days, and even now, don't go the extra mile and beg, really beg the question of why were those pets there in the first place?

The exploitation of animals is the subject of other books. The "Trap and Release" programs in many cities do try to address how we deal with feral cats and stray dogs that are not spayed or neutered. They are first trapped, then sterilized, then released back into their wild environment so that they cannot procreate and produce offspring. If the animals are not sterilized, their young is also free to reproduce with abandon, turning even more uncared for animals into the streets. It is a drop in a very large bucket, but it is more effective than doing nothing.

As technology improved and phones and cameras became smaller, documenting abuse became much easier. And very annoying for farmers, butchers and animal abusers who got caught red-handed with blood literally and figuratively on their hands on camera. Hence the passage in many states of "Ag Gag" laws which make it a felony to trespass, record and broadcast such truths. First amendment freedoms, freedom of the press and the future of our democracy is at risk, if these laws continue to be passed and enforced. If there is no accountability, leaders, corporations and their actions go unchecked and unquestioned. Even if these massive factory farms are on private property, the public has every right to know what goes on behind closed doors and just how badly many sentient beings are being brutally abused by heartless monsters. The public has every right to know what exactly they are paying someone else to do. The slaughtering, kicking and abusing of animals that have been so well recorded on smartphones and posted on social media, may very well be the job you or I would never do. How would we know what goes on behind closed doors if we didn't see it enough times on YouTube? The truth hurts. But we all need to see it and know it at some point so that we can make informed decisions how to spend our money and live our lives.

Evolution of Activism

Activism sometimes happens by accident. I remember the first time I heard someone introduce me at a talk as an activist. It caught me off guard. I had been a journalist for so long, and trained to get both sides of a story, no matter how difficult. I interviewed activists who I perceived to have an agenda with only one side of a story. That's just the way it was. But now, I realized, I had crossed the line and gone to the "dark side." But the only reason I did that was because I had seen all sides to the story. I had been gathering facts and information all my life, and the truth made me realize how much I needed to spend the rest of the my life getting the truth out there in real and meaningful ways. Finally, after so many years of trying to remain objective, I could cross the line and have an opinion. It was OK. It was more than OK. I feel and always will, that the future of our planet and all of our children depend on those willing to risk their livelihood, careers and even death threats to tell and show the truth.

Vegan Mythbusting

My publisher has asked me to write books every year, mainly because of the success of my first book, "Eat Vegan on $4 a Day." Every book I've written tackled and debunked long-held vegan myths. When my vegan sexual evolution and then revolution happened, my marketing maven brain started lighting up like a runner's endorphin high.

As much as I love my publisher, as I've mentioned, they didn't want me to write this vegan sex book with them. They were fine with my trying to get it done any way I could. Perhaps there was some reservation because vegan sex may not be the kind of book you can sell with children around, even if you put it in a brown wrapper. My marketing brain argued that as PETA's (People for the Ethical Treatment of Animals) Sexiest Vegan Over 50, who else is better qualified to write a book like this? Many people I spoke to about the working title, laughed and giggled, but they were very curious.

Because my publisher said "yes" to my first book "Eat Vegan on $4 a Day" when everybody else said no, I have always wanted to give them the first right of refusal on future books. I did believe in the vegan sex concept because I had been told by others I know in the book publishing industry that if you want a best-seller, write it about sex, money or murders, or better yet, some combination of the three.

I always thought trying to market a book based on sex was a little cheesy, and never wanted to stoop to what I previously believed were such low tactics. Then I realized that this is a really important topic with issues that haven't been brought to the forefront until now. I have been lucky to live a rich and fulfilling life. I have always viewed the world as my classroom. But it wasn't until I personally observed the difference between having sex or making love to a non-vegan and a vegan that my life changed forever. More people have to know how beautiful, rewarding and stimulating sex with a vegan can be, both in and out of bed. Sex, perhaps, is the last myth to fall by the wayside. I'm hoping. I would love for my mythbusting days to be over when the entire world connects the dots and we all become and remain committed to making the world a better, and truly compassionate and humane place. There was no question in my mind that this subject needed to come out from under the covers and see the light of day!

Workin' It: PETA, Marketing and Sex

I had been wanting to enter PETA's (People for the Ethical Treatment of Animals) "Sexiest Vegan Over 50" contest for years. It had nothing to do with looks, sexiness or sexuality. In fact, I had a chat with the 2016 Sexiest Vegan Over 50, Victoria Moran, who agreed with me that sexy, especially as we age when looks fade, is way more about vitality, enthusiasm and maintaining a positive outlook, as best you can in a crazy world. When I first broached the idea with an ex who had long-time erectile dysfunction, he immediately called me a slut for wanting to do such a thing. Suffice it to say, especially as a non-vegan, he just didn't get the whole animal rights picture, even though he had seen many of the movies and documentaries out at the time that detailed the horrific treatment of animals in our culture. I explained to him why I wanted to enter the contest. But it made no difference. If I had to point to the moment our relationship went south, that was it. This was where the thought that I gave up my marriage for veganism was born. But it was way more than that, as any break-up is. Growing in different directions? Perhaps. Some couples are able to grow together, even with major life changes occurring in the golden years. Many of us pay a huge price for our activism. But no matter. If it's the right thing to do, do it. Right?

Truth be known, my winning PETA's Sexiest Vegan Over 50 in 2014 was not at all about sex or looks. I, along with the many other candidates, and then finalists, were interviewed extensively by phone and in writing. After making the final cut of 10, there were many interviews, both written and verbal. PETA wanted to make sure if the media called, which they really haven't, I would be able to answer the many questions surrounding animal rights, and the necessary corollary: a vegan diet.

I laughed when several people asked me, "So...how many places has PETA sent you to all over the world, once you won this honor?" The truth is, zero. In fact, winners are asked to fly on their own dime for a professional photo shoot in Los Angeles donated by a local photographer, if they would like. Given that I lived in Florida, LA wasn't on my radar and I hired a local photographer to do a photo shoot. Point being, so many people have misconceptions about how the largest non-profits are rolling in the bucks. PETA's president, Ingrid Newkirk, takes a microscopic salary, as do many other animal rights and farm sanctuary activists and presidents. There's always a need for money to be spent on saving animals.

It didn't even occur to me at the time that I should fly to LA on my own dime to do a photoshoot, because I thought, having spent 18 years in the mainstream media, I knew how to write a news release. I knew how to call TV stations and get coverage. PETA wrote a great news release too, distributing it through the usual channels that TV, radio and print outlets check. The lack of a ringing phone was deafening. No money in broccoli. Victoria told me she actually hired a publicist for the only purpose of trying to arrange media interviews after she won. That was certainly beyond the call of duty and definitely not one of the job prerequisites. But upon further reflection, perhaps if I had thought to do that, I might have gotten at least one interview request. I suppose I should have known better. The media doesn't come crawling unless you're a drop-dead gorgeous celeb who lost 200 pounds. My 35 pound weight-loss seemed monumental to me for my 5 foot 3 body. So what that I'd placed in 100 at the time (as of this writing, it is 117) 5K or longer races for my age group, or was 7th in the US in the 1500 meters at the 2014 US National Senior Games. Nobody really cares. So what that I coached high school girls cross country and ran faster than most of the kids.

I had taught in all my years of media consulting that you have to take stories to the media on a silver platter. In my career, I heard constant criticism of the media, as I still do, that they don't do the right stories. They aren't mind readers. Hundreds or thousand of stories coming flying at them from all sources on a daily basis. And that's really the problem. News operations have closed all over the world from budget cutbacks. Covering serious news with inadequate resources is a serious problem. A news director or assignment or city editor can help filter, but not always. Corporate-driven agendas dictate what stories get done now more than ever. Corporate sponsors' money directs the focus or slant of too many news stories. When I was a mainstream reporter, that rarely, if ever happend. At most TV stations, and certainly every one I worked at, no one from the sales department was allowed to set foot in the newsroom. But that was a long time ago.

Always. Listen. To. Your. Heart.

I'd held off entering PETA's contest for several years fearing I would anger my ex. I mentioned my thoughts about entering to no one except my ex. When I got a call asking me to enter, I said, "You know, this is a great organization that does valuable undercover investigations which cost money, both in time, staff, resources and potentially fighting expensive lawsuits. By fighting the AG Gag laws as they do, they are really fighting for freedom of the press." I thought that might win him over. He still threw barbs my way.

So I quietly slunk away and figured I'll just enter and probably won't win against stiff competition.

I thought that the odds were not great of my becoming a finalist or actually winning. What could possibly go wrong? Except that I did win.

My ex was not happy. Not happy at all. He called me a slut. Again. But this time with hateful vengeance. The handwriting was on the wall. Again.

The real reason I entered the contest was because I learned a long time ago back in my early reporting days that animal rights stories never got coverage unless PETA asked a couple of gorgeous scantily clad volunteers to wear fake furs in the middle of January protesting in front of a fur store. They knew how to work the media and what would draw in the journalists and the cameras. They knew the visuals sold. I was the reporter covering those stories. It wasn't up to me whether those stories saw the light of day. It was all about what management wanted, usually all male management.

Why else did I want to enter the contest? Because for years, people have questioned my age, commenting I look so much younger than I am. In a discussion with other female vegan authors, we came to discover that we have received this same kind of feedback over the ages. And as we age, the demands to know how we do what we do to "look like that" increase. People are always looking for the fountain of youth. An antioxidant, plant-rich, plant-pure, plant-exclusive or whatever you want to call it gives you that glow, especially the closer you get to nature and the least processed foods sneak into your diet.

The Natural Foods Expo, a mega double-wide mammoth convention center site in Anaheim, California, is the mecca for new products sold to any health food store in America. Increasingly, the food companies are finding ways to grab the vegan market, and anyone who has money to buy those products. As one of my friends who attended said, "I had a really tough time finding broccoli, or any fresh foods. We had to go to the grocery store." So sometimes, less is more.

What is a vegan diet, in case you're new here? Nothing with a mother or a face. Or as some of the staunchest animal rights activists say, it is not just a diet. It is a lifestyle. It is a way of life. It is a mindset where you don't buy, use and especially exploit animals in any way. So no meat product consumption at all. No eggs. No dairy. Not even stressing bees by imposing our human desires to take their honey, even if it is "good" for them. Which it isn't. Some activists say that even the word "exploit" is too vague and wishy-washy. We should be using the words that most and best describe what happens to animals: rape, murder, tortured, abused, mutilated, or kidnapped. If you don't have the visual on that yet, go directly to YouTube and search "factory farms in the US." Or watch "Dairy is Scary." It is 5 minutes of the most powerful and well-edited videos that will get you up to speed on all the issues in no time. Every time I post this link on Facebook, at least 2 or 3 people comment that they are now done with dairy and are so thankful to have learned from the video.

When I taught cooking classes for a vegan animal rights and health-focused national non-profit just after the turn of the century, (oh...that sounds like a long time ago) we were told to drop the "v" or vegan word, and replace it with "plant-based." The organization wanted to remove the association of animal rights with veganism and turn the national attention to eating a vegan diet as much for health, or even more so than any other reason. It worked. The testimonials poured in from our classes with so many people from the mainstream who would have never before considered a vegan diet for losing weight, reducing their A1C numbers for diabetes, and even reversing cancer, as described earlier with a multiple myeloma cancer survivor. Yes, we must avoid saying that a vegan diet is the sure cure for cancer. But it sure helps so many people as the many vegan doctor heroes have documented.

"Plant-Based" VS "Vegan"

If you Google "plant-based," my interview with the Tampa Bay times in 2011, is the first reference to the concept of replacing the "v" word with "plant-based" to break out of the animal rights association with veganism. But the more that videos surface documenting the abuse so many of us saw decades ago, more of us are feeling less apologetic and are instead, embracing our inner and outer veganism and activism. For me, activism takes form on many platforms, from social media to crossing a 5K finish line in a vegan shirt. It's all good, however you define it. I encourage you to find your inner activist and do what feels right. The bottom line is getting to the point where you no longer want to use or exploit animals in any form or fashion. You have seen the light and are totally born again. Oh we are sounding a little cultish, aren't we now? So be it.

Traumatized Into Veganism

My journey to veganism began when my aunt died of breast cancer in our home when I was 5. Relatives were wailing, my 6 year-old cousin who was now motherless, came to live with us and would sob and rock herself to sleep every night for the next year. Trauma doesn't even begin to describe it. As I watched my mom and both sisters eventually get breast cancer, and all the other diseases of affluence...heart disease, diabetes, Alzheimer's and the "minor" conditions like arthritis, macular degeneration and varicose veins, I would soon learn and believe that most of their diseases were totally preventable. Because of our family history of breast cancer, we became part of the original breast cancer gene studies, although no one in our family needed a study to tell us what we already knew--that we had the gene. 4 people in one immediate -family with breast cancer? That was pretty high and rare. Interestingly, because of confidentiality, the studies don't let you know if you have the gene. But for the rest of my life or until the Affordable Care Act no longer made it an pre-existing condition should I get cancer, I would lead my life as if I had the gene. I would learn from genetic counselors that 2 of the 4 breast cancer cases in my family were most likely genetic since they occurred when the women were in their 30's--very early. The other two cases were late in life, so those are suspected of being environmentally caused. The study of epigenetics is all about that--what genes are turned on or off by our lifestyle choices.

As an Emmy-winning TV investigative reporter for 18 years in Miami and St. Louis, figuring out how to avoid our family scourges became the investigative reporting job of my life. It was in the TV newsroom where at the age of 28, I collapsed and almost died of a colon blockage. Two colleagues "piled" me and my "piles" (another word for inflamed hemorrhoids caused by chronic constipation) into a car and drove me to the emergency room where doctors said they had never seen a blockage that large in someone my age, and that I would need to be on medicine the rest of my life to prevent that from happening again.

I ran to the hospital and read all 5 books on fiber, because that's all there was at the time. The research and writings of Denis Burkitt blew my eyes wide open as I realized that in some places of the world, mainly Africa, where primitive high-fiber diets were commonplace, that bowel movements were as frequent as 3 a day. In my world, 3 a week were cause for celebration.

I started by simply adding loose bran fiber to my cereals and was blown away by how just that, along with moving to a high-fiber diet rich in vegetables, fruits and whole grains made all the difference in the world. Like many my age, I first began with a macrobiotic diet which was basically vegan, except that it included white fish and all kinds of difficult to follow rules such as eating only foods in your latitude (so oranges and grapefruits from Florida were nixed in Missouri). I felt great eating that way, especially with the addition of nutrient-rich varieties of seaweed and miso soup. But it was hard to find brown rice vegetable sushi in the drive throughs on the way back from stories, if we even had time to do that. Unfortunately, restaurants, especially fast food restaurants, were not at all vegan friendly back then, except for maybe french fries. And often, they were deep fried in animal fat.

Vegetarian books exploded on the market with the likes of "Laurel's Kitchen" and Dr. Neal Barnard's first books. "The Power of Your Plate" which shared the opinions of the doctors who did the first open heart surgeries.

Excited as they were to be on the forefront of new medical technology, they quickly realized and said, if you do all these great procedures but don't change your diet, you'll be back on the operating table in a year's time. How prophetic that would become. The leap from vegetarianism which still included eggs and dairy to veganism which excluded them, was not quite as rapid. Books and events that were really 100% vegan were still titled "vegetarian," and to some extent, events such as North American Vegetarian Summerfest and "veggiefests" which are events designed to attract newbies to the food, issues and causes involved with a vegan diet and lifestyle, still hang on to the "vegetarian" word. Old habits are hard to die. There is something to be said for using the larger, broader-encompassing word to gather more people into the fold before dumping the "v" word on them. Others, such as the vegan feminist agitator, as she likes to be known, and organizer of the fabulous monster event, "Chicago Veganmania," Marla Rose, makes no apologies for calling her gathering a vegan event, and nothing but.

Our culture is steeped in dancing around issues with euphemistic words. With my family history of breast cancer, I had doctors telling me at an early age, even before I was married, to consider breastfeeding because it was known to be preventative against breast cancer, not only in moms, but in female offspring as research would later prove. In short, considering the heart disease, diabetes, morbid obesity, Alzheimer's and high blood pressure in our family, doctors bluntly said, "You better do something differently or you will end up like everybody else in your family." I began searching like there was no tomorrow.

My obstetrician almost apologetically told me during one of my exams after I was pregnant, "You might want to check out a group called La Leche League. They're kind of militant, but they know their stuff." While that was the reputation the group had, especially in the mainstream, nothing could have been farther from the truth. The legend of La Leche League developed in its infancy when the 6 courageous founding mothers wanted to form a breastfeeding information and support group because nowhere in American culture could women view other women breastfeeding. Not knowing or seeing how to do it, was the number one reason for failure. So the group, somewhat challenged by the concept, and not necessarily wanting to utter the word "breast" or publically talk about a group that used the word "breast," they came up with "La Leche," which is Spanish for "the milk."

I found the groups to be welcoming, educational and informative. I was incredibly motivated to learn as much as I could about our own species' specific milk and to do everything I could to avoid failure. After all, one of my older sisters had breastfed each of her 4 children for 6 months a piece and still got breast cancer. The handwriting was on the wall that I was going to have to take this little endeavor seriously. I knew I had to succeed not only for my own avoidance of breast cancer...use it or lose it...but for the sake of my three daughters. Genetic odds are, one of the four of us would get breast cancer, and I was determined to do everything I could to try to keep from turning on those genes, if in fact, I or they had them.

I not only joined La Leche League, but I became an accredited leader and then took on a statewide leadership position as the associate coordinator of leader applicants for Missouri. Any member wanting to become a leader would have to submit a written application answering many questions. It was my decision as to whether a mom would become a leader or not. For the most part, it was self-selecting. Anyone who submitted an application really wanted the volunteer job and knew that their role would mean answering those middle of the night calls, "My baby won't nurse. Help!"

Known as a gutsy former TV reporter who quit her job to be a stay-at-home mom for 6 years, leaving "the best job in local television," according to my general manager, I was often asked to speak on panels at local, state and national conferences on "Having it all, but not all at the same time." Given that I was a child of the 60's who fought for women's rights in high school and college, I had vowed I would always work and not give in to those hormones that so many women described when they quit their jobs after giving birth to stay home with their babies. No, I would never do that.

Then I learned about hormones. They made me quit my job. I learned how women's eyes dilate when they see a baby. Any baby. Not just their own. Even babies in other species. No wonder we coo at bunnies and can't imagine how they are used increasingly now for meat consumption. But human mothers especially coo loudest with their own babies who seem to cast magical spells. The general manager's words slid off of me like oil. I taught pre-school. I dusted off my guitar and was a songleader. I had an organic garden, cooked from scratch every day and even made homemade bread, until the bread-maker caught on fire. I probably used too much whole wheat which overtaxed the motor. I wasn't the perfect earth mother kneading by hand. But I did manage to stay home for 6 years until my ex lost his job and I had to go back to work. What I learned was that bonding doesn't happen in a vacuum. Quality time doesn't happen without a lot quantity time. As much as I wanted to believe differently, and even worked part-time during the first year after my oldest child was born, it wasn't the same as being there full-time.

The days of setting up the first women's center at the University of Missouri while managing a journalism degree, becoming the first woman to anchor the evening news at the university's station which, at the time was the only traditional, commercial network affiliate licensed to a university board of curators, seemed light years away. When I got my journalism degree, the ratio of women to men was 1 to 5. Women were still struggling and trying to smash glass ceilings. Some thought they had to get to the top on their back. I refused. But mine was the first generation of women that could even entertain the idea. I was willing to put that all on hold when my children were young, until I had to go back to work.

After I wrote "Eat Vegan on $4 a Day," I realized that there was no money in broccoli and that I would have to use my investigative skills to really dig deep into the research and news stories of the day to separate out facts from fiction. I would ask who funded the studies and try to discover whose names kept recurring in studies that were covertly funded by meat and dairy interests. The connecting of dots between the health of animals, the planet, a healthful diet to hopefully avoid disease while enhancing a budding athletic performer who only recently discovered her inner track star genes, had just begun. Most of us were not born into vegan families. We all started somewhere. It is important for all of us to remember this when trying to help others on their journey. Sometimes, we become so impatient and even angry that the world, our friends, and especially our relatives aren't moving at light speed. You can lead a horse to water, but you can't make it drink. You must live and breathe the example you want others to become.

As animal activist Rae Sikora is fond of saying, you don't have a choice in your birth family. But you do have a choice in your chosen family. Choose wisely. Channel the animals.

CHAPTER 3

The Research on Heart Disease and What It Means to Erectile Dysfunction

Of Hard Attacks and Heart Attacks: Why Does a Cardiologist Care?

Why would a cardiologist care about the quality of your erection? Your ejaculation? Your orgasm? Is it appropriate for a university professor to write about topics usually under cover or in brown wrappers? Actually, the history and science of sex has been intertwined with heart and artery health for decades. And although not all sex is driven by emotions of love, the symbol of the heart for love has to be regarded as tying the pillow and the pump together.

Take for example the pill that changed male behavior forever. While you might be thinking the birth control pill which did have a profound impact on increasing sexual activity, I am referring to the blue pill known as Viagra. Viagra, or sildenafil in its generic form, was not intended to make men better in the sack. It was identified as a compound that had favorable effects on arteries and was tested by the giant pharmaceutical house Pfizer for the treatment of high blood pressure and heart disease. In one of the most memorable series of side effect reported by these men, a new chapter in sex was written. While the patients in these early trials reported some improvement in cardiac function, they also testified to tighter pants, easier erections, and greater success in completing the sex act. For many of these men with cardiovascular disease this was the first time in a long while that the fire below was hot enough to raise the flag pole and they were ecstatic about continuing the drug. Pfizer sensed a winning drug of another kind and shifted the trials to sexual success. The approval process for the drug known as Viagra proceeded and was approved by the FDA in 1998. This soon became a multibillion dollar drug. To bring the complete the circle of history to the current era, Viagra has recently been studied in Sweden and the results were presented at a national cardiology meeting this year. In 43,000 men who had suffered a first heart attack, the usage of any of the family of erectile dysfunction drugs, including Viagra, Cialis and Levitra, was observed to reduce the risk of dying of any cause by 33% over the 3.3-year study interval. That might be a big advantage to the survivor of a heart attack and is gratifying to know the safety of sex in general and these drugs in particular. Surely, further study is needed. For now, it appears more blood to the wood is good for heart and soul.

Why does a drug that is good for heart arteries prove to be good for the wood too? Is there a link between the sexual response of men and women and cardiovascular health? Actually, there is a very strong connection between arteries and sex organs as all sex organs (a very dry term for your junk) are supplied by arteries. Taking care of your heart and arteries may be the best sex aid ever. Almost 400 years ago, English physician Thomas Sydenham wrote that "a man is as old as his arteries." The modern version would be "men, women and trans-genders are as old as their arteries" or as I like to spin it positive "you are as young as your arteries." Put one more way, 'you are as hard as your arteries are soft." My cardiology practice is dedicated to helping arteries stay young for health and longevity. Successful and vigorous sex is a part of many people's definition of health so it is all intertwined. Every day I ask all of my male patients about their ability to develop and maintain an erection. Although the usual response is "strong like bull," many men do have serious problems.

Can erectile dysfunction in a man develop as a sign of sick arteries before a life threatening heart attack or stroke? YES, and this is so important to know and seek a full evaluation if the penis is not responding like it used to. While I am certain this is true for women too, there is just about no data so forgive me the male orientation to the discussion. Recent data indicate that identifying a man with diabetes who is unable to have a satisfactory erection can predict the presence of diseased arteries and future heart events several years before a heart attack or heart death (https://www.ncbi.nlm.nih.gov/m/ pubmed/22962586/?i=6&from=erectile%2520dysfunction%2520preficts% 2520CV%2520disease). The predictive power of erectile dysfunction on heart events is even more powerful than asking about smoking, blood pressure, or even a family history of early heart attacks.

If you have erectile dysfunction, or sleep with a man that does, getting to the doctor for a complete evaluation may allow time to identify, treat, and reverse arterial damage before bad things happen. Do yourself or your man a favor and share this information in a supportive way. Teaching more people about the data indicating that there is "survival of the firmest" could save many lives. All you have to do is practice a lifestyle that promotes arterial health, head-to-toe, but with emphasis on the joy of the groin. Let's learn a bit more about the linkage between the groin-heart connection.

1.   Why is there a connection between healthy arteries and successful sex?

There are 50,000 miles of arteries coursing through our bodies although guys are mainly concerned with about 6 inches, not miles. Inside every artery is an inner lining that is only one cell layer thick that is called the endothelium. An appreciation of the role of the endothelium for health was so significant that three researchers were awarded the Nobel Prize in Medicine in 1998 for this finding. They docs figured out that when the endothelium is healthy it produces a gas called nitric oxide (NO). This is different from nitrous oxide known as laughing gas. Arteries can make a lot of NO or just a little. When a lot of NO is produced, arteries relax allowing more blood flow and more normal blood pressure, resists plaque and clogging up, and resist blood clots that cause heart attack and stroke. It turns out, to have a great sex response, lots of blood brought in by lots of NO is needed to swell the necessary tissues. Endothelial dysfunction (ED), or dicksfunction if you want to make people laugh, leads to a poor blood flow response throughout the body and poor maintenance of the swollen penis needed to create and sustain an erection. Say just say Yes to NO.

2.   What harms your endothelium?

How many times have you heard that eating fruits and vegetables can improve your health? Do you do it? If you do, you are in the 1.5% of Americans that actually practice what I preach regarding healthy eating. If you include the healthy habits of eating well, not smoking, exercising regularly, and maintaining a proper weight, only 3% of Americans go 4 for 4 on that measurement. These are the very lifestyle factors that are known to harm the endothelium and its production of NO. Do you like to smoke? You will make less NO. Do you like to sit and watch movies? You will make less NO. Do you like to eat fast food and gain weight? You will make less NO. Do you like donuts more than grapes? You will make less NO. Lifestyles decisions can lead to hypertension, diabetes, elevated cholesterol and obesity and all can produce erectile and endothelial dysfunction by the production of less NO.

The standard American diet is high in processed foods packed with chemicals, fat, sugar and salt and is often combined with a sedentary lifestyle, poorly managed stress, intake of environmental toxins like plastic bottles made from bisphenol A (BPA), and poor sleep. These are all factors that produce reduce NO and produce ED. Diets emphasizing plant-powered rainbow foods, naturally low fats and rich in minerals, vitamins, phytonutrients promote arterial health and erectile success. These are the NO boosters. Next time you see your produce managers at the grocery store or farmer's market, give them the respect they deserve as sexual counselors.

3.   How powerful a predictor is erectile dysfunction for silent heart disease?

ED is a powerful predictor of future coronary artery disease events. For example, if you live in Olmsted County, Minnesota and are a man between the ages of 40 and 49 without known heart disease but with ED, you have up to a 50-fold higher incidence of eventually having new heart events compared to men the same age without ED (https://www.ncbi.nlm.nih. gov/pubmed/19181643). Rarely in medicine is there ever a risk factor this powerful. (By comparison, smoking may raise your risk of similar events 3-fold. Please do not smoke.)

4.   What do you do if you have erectile dysfunction?

Although this is a book on vegan sex, not Vegan Cardiology, my passion is both to spread the love of plant based health and early heart disease detection. When ED is an issue, even if an early issue that was not present before, my advice is to see a physician, perhaps a cardiologist, interested in advanced detection and prevention of arteries. This may not be so simple as some doctors in primary care, cardiology and urology sadly are not aware of the established connection between the heart bone and boning. This is unfortunate as there are extensive medical articles written on the topic that are available to all healthcare professionals. The most exhaustive medical reference is the Princeton III Consensus Recommendations for the Management of Erectile Dysfunction and Cardiovascular Disease (https://www.ncbi.nlm.nih.gov/pmc/articles/PMC3498391/pdf/main.

pdf). In my preventive cardiology office, I see patients who come solely for evaluation of their ED with no known heart issues. Most will have problems with blood pressure, cholesterol, blood sugar, family history of heart disease or obesity, or all of the above, to make the visit simpler to fit into standard office billing diagnoses. The patients I see are going to receive instructions to address their diet, exercise, and stress management as I educate and guide them to an artery healthy lifestyle that promotes a strong heart, rich production of NO, and a strong erection. All of the "numbers" that matter for cardiovascular health will be measured. These can include blood pressure, weight, waist circumference, fasting blood sugar and insulin, total cholesterol and LDL particle number, hs-CRP for inflammation, homocysteine for methylation, and lpa or lipoprotein a (an inherited form of cholesterol that can clog arteries but is rarely measured). An EKG will be performed.

As ED can be a clue to silent but serious heart artery blockages, I will usually go a step further than just the numbers above. Generally, I recommend patients have a coronary artery calcium scan (CACS) using a modern high-speed CT scanner at a local hospital that generally costs under $200. You may have never heard of this test but it has been around for over 15 years and has thousands of medical research papers supporting it as the most accurate way to determine if the heart arteries are young, medium or old. It is a simple CT scan over the heart without and IV, iodine dye, or injection. There is a fascinating documentary called The Widowmaker about how this test was developed. Old heart arteries, even if silent in terms of symptoms, are calcified heart arteries, and they show up on the CT scan reliably. The whole test takes under a minute and results in a score that should be Zero. If you want to score for a long time, you want a heart CT score of zero. This means that the ED is not due to advanced silent heart blockages. That is great news. If the number is high, and it can be 200 or 2,000 even in active people assuming they are healthy inside, then a protocol to halt and reverse heart disease with lifestyle and integrative measures can be implemented.

Only recently can we approximate NO production by a simple blood test. It is not known to most doctors and not available in all labs but in my clinic I will measure the level of ADMA. When this compound is high it means NO production is low. When it is low, it means NO production is normal and high. It can also change quickly from abnormal to normal when a better diet, exercise, smoking cessation, and stress management are implemented along with some supplements like L-arginine. In addition, there is now a way to directly measure the health of the endothelium and its production of NO. This is called an EndoPAT examination and is like a very fancy blood pressure cuff. In my office I perform this non-invasive test on men with ED to see if their endothelium is acting healthy or sick. I then make a program for better arteries and better sex and recheck it in a few months.

To wrap up the topic of the connection between sex and the health of your heart, let's talk about a canary. In case you have never heard this piece of mining lore, a trick used by miners to avoid being exposed to and dying from elevated levels of toxic gases was to bring a caged canary into the coal mine. If the canary acted strange or died the miners knew to exit the mine immediately before they were at risk for death because the bird suffered effects of the gases before the larger workers. Erectile dysfunction is often referred to as a canary in the coal mine. The erection that doesn't happen or cannot be sustained can give clues to poor lifestyles and sick arteries 3 to 4 years before the heart attack strikes. Just like the miners fleeing the mine, you should run to a health care professional familiar with endothelium, NO and ED and get an check-up. You might save a life and restore sexual performance and joy.

CHAPTER 4

Physiology of Sex and Food: Vegans, Vaginas, Vegetables, and Vas Deferens

Hot, sweaty passionate love up and down a staircase like The Thomas Crown Affair…all happens because your mindset is right and your arteries and heart are acting youthful. Is vegan sex really the best sex in terms of the science of food and fornication? While there has been a lot of bravado and testimonials about the enhanced sexual prowess, longevity, taste and general sexiness of those following a plant-based diet, does the science support it? One of the most famous of the testimonials to vegan vigor in bed is found in the movie Forks Over Knives (www.forksoverknives.com). If you have never seen this classic, please watch it. In this hit documentary, reference is made to the ability to "raise the flag" on a plant-based diet even in patients with advanced heart disease. PETA (People for the Ethical Treatment of Animals) has contributed to the banter with sexy ads submitted to the Super Bowl but banned as they were just too steamy. They declared "Go Vegan, Last Longer" and you can find the short You Tube on the web some night when kids have gone to bed early. In the scientific arena there is every reason to believe from a medical viewpoint that vegan sex is the most reliable pathway to male and female potency and performance for as long as possible.

Maybe you are wondering why you need to learn more about the physiology of sex and veganism if it is all working successfully for you. The sad truth is that there is such a high rate of problems with sexual performance that planning for the future is a smart plan even if you are a Tarzan or Jane right now. Indeed, your spoon can help you spoon far into the future.

There is more science to the sequence of events creating an erection than there is for the female counterpart so here is a brief and graphic rundown on how it all happens. If you are a visual learner and want a laugh out loud experience learning about this, just Google Woody Allen's "Everything You Wanted to Know About Sex" from 1972 and look up the sperm scene. Here is the drier version.

1) Touch, sights, sounds, erotic memories, and fantasies cause sexual excitement.

2) These stimuli increase signal output from a part of the brain called the para-ventricular nucleus. I love this part of the brain.

3) These signals then pass through special autonomic nerves in the spinal cord, the pelvic nerves and the cavernous nerves that run along the prostate gland to reach the corpora cavernosa and the arteries that supply them with blood.

4) In response to these signals, the muscle fibers in the corpora cavernosa relax, allowing blood to fill the spaces within them if the endothelium is healthy.

5) Muscle fibers in the arteries that supply the penis also relax, and there is an eight-fold increase in blood flow to the penis. The increased blood flow expands the sinusoidal spaces in the corpora, then stretches the surrounding sheath.

6) As the tunica stretches, it blocks off the veins that take blood away from the corpora cavernosa. This traps blood within the penis, the pressure becomes very high and the penis becomes erect. This is ingenious. Let the red blood in and cut of the escape hatch for the blood in the veins.

7) During an erection pressure in the penis is at least twice the pressure of blood in the main circulation. This is possible because the muscles of the pelvic floor contract around the base of the corpora cavernosa.

8) At orgasm, the signaling from the brain changes dramatically. There is a sudden increase in norepinehphrine (adrenaline) production from nerves in the genitalia. This seems to both trigger orgasm and contract the muscle fibers in the corpora cavernosa and their supplying arteries. As a result of this the blood flow into the penis reduces.

9) The pressure within the corpora drops, which also relaxes the tunica and so allows blood to flow out of the penis. This allows the penis to become flaccid again. This is when some smoke a cigarette but I advise against this Hollywood habit.

How big a problem is the penis that won't stay big? There are an estimated 30 million men in the U.S. alone with erectile dysfunction (ED) and the problem is growing while the male organ is not. When sexual function falters, not only may romantic life suffer but overall health and specifically heart health can suffer too. As you now know, research shows that ED can be an early warning sign of heart disease. Words like "sorry, I do not know what is wrong but it is just not working like it used to" can forewarn the coming of a heart attack 3-4 years in the future when nothing else is coming. Is it a coincidence that two medical terms of interest, endothelial dysfunction (poor artery health) and erectile dysfunction (limpus penosus) are both abbreviated ED? In fact, if you want to be good in the BED, you do not want either ED in your life. When there is ED (erectile dysfunction) there is ED (endothelial dysfunction) to blame. Healthy arteries are FUNdamental for a good firm arousal and for all swollen parts in both genders. Around 300 years ago, Ben Franklin wrote that an ounce of prevention is worth a pound of cure. Similarly, I tell my male patients "to be older and hard, exercise daily and eat no lard!" Let's turn to some research on the relationship between dietary choices and successful sex vegan style that you may use.

The Sexiest Foods Are Plant-Based

Researchers from Harvard Medical School performed the first observational study of dietary habits and sexual function over a 10-year period so you can pick foods for frolicking fun. The authors of the study estimated that over 300 million men worldwide will soon suffer from erectile dysfunction and that vascular disease, or sick blood vessels, was a common cause linking ED to heart disease and stroke. These scientists conducted a prospective study among 25,096 men from the Health Professionals Follow-Up Study. The study concentrated on how many servings these men were eating of plant-based foods, particularly those plant foods rich in flavonoid compounds known to be favorable to artery health. While foods in grocery stores are not labeled flavonoids, some of the foods you are buying or growing already are rich in these sexy compounds. These include strawberries, blueberries, apples, pears, and citrus foods like lemons and limes. Participants gave details of their diet every 4 years and rated their erectile function in 2000, 2004 and again in 2008 (no pictures were required to be sent in). During 10 years of follow-up of these health professionals, a sobering 36% of the men reported erectile dysfunction. It appears being a doctor is not a guarantee of being immune to impotence. It also makes you wonder about taking advice on nutrition from many health professionals who have little education in the field and suffer the same consequences of the standard American diet that the rest of the population suffer. After analyzing additional factors known to be harmful to arteries supplying the sex organs, such as smoking, diabetes, and high cholesterol, several specific foods were associated with less ED, better erections, and better sex. The higher the intake of foods rich in the family of flavonoid compounds (flavanones, anthocyanins, and flavones), the lower the risk of ED. If you remember only one lesson on eating for sexual health, the higher the intake of fruit, the lower the risk of erectile dysfunction. To have a banana, eat a banana and such examples. Indeed, men eating the most fruit had a 14% reduction in risk of ED over the 10 years. It appears that if you add fruit today you can keep the blue pill away. The Harvard data showed that eating strawberries, blueberries, apples, pears, and citrus products instead of chips, cookies and fries, can maintain normal sexual responsiveness. I recommend you make a firm commitment to eating more plant-based foods, particularly fruit, no matter how hard.

Everyone appreciates how sexy the Europeans are with their body fitting clothes, free spirit about nude beaches, and acceptance of sex as a normal human function. It may be worth looking at some medical data from Europe we can use to maintain our sexual prowess. Professor Esposito of Naples, Italy has done a series of studies on the Mediterranean diet (MED) and erectile dysfunction. The MED diet is a very plant-strong model to study and there are versions that are "vegiterranean" and include only plant based foods. In one study by Dr. Esposito, the effect of a Mediterranean-style diet on ED in men was examined (3). All the men had a syndrome called the metabolic syndrome combining abdominal obesity, high triglycerides, low HDL cholesterol, a high blood pressure, and an elevated blood sugar that together predicts increased cardiac risk. Sixty-five men with both ED and the metabolic syndrome met the criteria. Half of them were assigned to the Mediterranean-style diet and 30 to the control diet. After 2 years, men on the Mediterranean diet consumed more fruits, vegetables, nuts, whole grain, and olive oil as compared with men on the control diet. Blood tests indicating healthy arteries improved in the MED diet group and were unchanged in the control group. There were 13 men in the intervention group and two in the control group that reported improved sexual function measures. The study overall suggested that a Mediterranean-style diet rich in whole grains, fruits, vegetables, legumes, walnut, and olive oil might be effective in reducing the prevalence of ED in men with the metabolic syndrome. I am confident adding these foods to anyone with ED, whether they have the diagnosis of metabolic syndrome or not, would help their ability to experience the joy of sex. The power of food to prevent and heal damaged endothelium and create more NO can result in better sexual responsiveness within just a few weeks.

How consistent is the data that the plant-based components of the MED diet may boost sexual performance? In a series of 440 patients studied in Spain, there were 42% that reported ED (4). Factors related to ED were studied in terms of diet, lifestyle and other factors. Patients with ED were more frequently smokers, sedentary, and consumed more alcohol. Eating nuts and vegetables lowered the risk of ED by about half. Obesity, heart disease, and steady alcohol consumption were directly related to ED. Overall, erectile dysfunction was a very common disorder in these patients treated in Spain with risk factors for heart disease. Eating vegetables and nuts may be protective and are known to heal endothelium and drive NO production to higher levels.

The reason plant-based foods can quickly boost sexual function takes us back to endothelium and NO production. The pathways by which NO is produced in the endothelium of arteries, whether in the groin or the heart, led to the awarding of the Nobel Prize in Medicine in 1998. The amino acids L-arginine and L-citrulline cycle back and forth and create NO in endothelial cells. This system is particularly active before the age of 40. A smart plan to maintain high sexual performance is to eat foods high in L-arginine that lead to NO production. If you be sure to eat occasional pine nuts, peanuts, walnuts, almonds, pistachios, and Brazil nuts you will be getting L-arginine in your diet. If you are watching your weight, and who isn't, be sure you limit nuts to about a small handful a day as they are calorie dense. Whole grains, like oats and wheat germ, also have significant amounts of L-arginine and are a healthy part of any diet.

Earlier I mentioned the amino acid L-citrulline. This is another amino acid found in foods that can help arteries be responsive to support romance and passion. Where do you find L-citrulline? Watermelon has the highest concentration of citrulline in nature (particularly the white rind) and yellow watermelon is higher than red brands. L-citrulline is also found in onions and garlic. Watermelon might be a better choice however before going on a date!

In addition to eating foods rich in L-arginine and L-citrulline to provide the building block for NO production, there is second way to generate NO. There are chemicals called dietary nitrates found in many foods like greens and beets that can be converted in our saliva to nitrites, absorbed, and then converted to NO. You can actually chew cruciferous vegetables and end up with the same reaction you might get from a prescription medication, more NO! Because this reaction requires healthy mouth bacteria found in grooves in our tongues, you can interrupt the process by using antiseptic mouthwashes. These products can kill helpful bacteria and prevent healthy conversion of dietary nitrates to nitrites leading to NO production and successful sex.

The cruciferous vegetables that are rich in dietary nitrates include arugula, rhubarb, kale Swiss chard, spinach, and bok choy. Beets and the beetroot can also supply dietary nitrates whether they are eaten or juiced. Beet off takes on a new meaning when you understand NO production. By adding grapes, pomegranates, apples and green teas to your diet you have a dynamite erotic potion.

Women also need blood flow for romance and the same systems work in the female body although they are studied less often in research protocols. There are limited studies using drugs like Viagra in women with diabetes and sexual dysfunction and benefits were reported. As the mechanism by which Viagra leads to sexual improvement has the same end result as the NO pathways, it is reasonable to suspect that women eating foods rich in L-arginine, L-citrulline and dietary nitrates will experience a boost in their sexual responsiveness too.

Overall, men often like to brag about their sexual prowess, whether in the gym or the bedroom. This bragging is often somehow tied up with eating steaks, smoking cigars, and watching football for hours while sitting on the couch, all activities likely to lead to less NO and more ED. In my opinion, the sexist man is the one who loves animals but does not eat them and who takes care of his health by getting exercise and not smoking. This is true of women too. While more research is needed, the best blue pill is a blueberry. The best aphrodisiac is a person in tune with kindness to animals, the confidence knowing the environment is suffering as little as possible by wise plant-based food choices made, and enjoying the sexual benefits of plant-powered genitals.

For full disclosure, a diet loaded with whole food plants in place of animals based foods may not reverse or protect every single example of ED and female sexual dysfunction. Sorry, but if someone guarantees you a 100% result, run the other way. Sex is simply too complicated. Even though sex is dependent on a brisk and healthy system of blood flow redirection for the erection and female climax, it is also has some components that even arugula and watermelon may not fix. We have learned a lot about the sexual response from the American research team of Masters and Johnson and their seminal work (awkward word choice) in the 1960s. They described stages of the sexual response and not all of them, particularly the fifth one, will smooth out with a smoothie. In fact, I think the best analogy to the Masters and Johnson formula is a smoothie. If you do not want to make one at all (Stage 5), why bother with the rest of the stages. But if you do, you need some interest (Stage 1, arousal), some rather cumbersome planning of cutting and prepping (Stage 2, plateau), activating the button (Stage 3, Orgasm), and the deceleration (Stage 4, Resolution). Let's take our knowledge of making smoothies and blasts and apply it to the stages of your vegan sexual journey.

Stage 1: Arousal

This stage of sex is characterized by a rapid, sometimes super rapid, response of the penis and female tissues to any and all excitement from visual stimuli (i.e. ogling), physical stimuli (like holding hands, kissing or grinding pelvic structures together on the dance floor), or psychological stimuli (like loving emotions which I am told by others may work if there is enough alcohol involved). As you know, arteries will dilate and blood flow will increase permitting swelling of sexual tissues with blood as manifested most obviously by the erect penis. This is one stage that lifestyle and healthy eating will enhance.

During this stage there is an increase in the heart rate and blood pressure if the cardiovascular system is healthy and unencumbered by medications. Although this may sound like a lot of wiring and plumbing, this stage may happen in as short as 30 seconds, particularly if a Michael Buble or a Barry White song is playing. With age, medical conditions or prescription drugs, the arousal stage may result in slower changes.

The Second Stage: Plateau

Now that everything is swollen, wet and primed for action, it would be a good time to remove some clothing or at least push some aside. With continued stimulation and no interference (cell phones, dogs, cats, children of any age, doorbells, work deadlines, to do lists, unusual body odors, misplaced body hairs, gas, itching…there can be a lot of distractions), the testicles will lift toward the body, the penis reaches full erection, and the number of breaths per minute peak in the 30's to 40's per minute. The healthier the heart and arteries, the easier this stage will be so eat wisely.

Premature ejaculation can interrupt this stage in a man and the key is to achieve control over this plateau stage. A yoga practice concentrating on core strength is one of the exercises that can be practiced in order to achieve control over early ejaculation. And as many yogis are vegan, we are back to your diet again.

The Third Stage – Orgasm

This is a short stage but I am hopeful that genetic engineering or stem cell transplants may extend this stage to hours or weeks (like the Orgasmatron in another Woody Allen classic, Sleeper). Orgasm happens with the rhythmic contractions nearly every second of genital muscles spreading to the entire body including the overall sensation of the big O.

For men, orgasm includes ejaculation. Fatigue, alcohol, or prescription medications or someone knocking on the door are all reasons that a man may find it difficult to finish up ejaculate. It is possible that foods that diminish the health of arteries, even briefly, may prevent a successful erection and ejaculation. The Big Mac Attack, for example, may indeed attack a man's ability to perform and leave him looking like Ronald the clown.

The convulsions of muscles during orgasms, which are initially strong and then weaker dammit, are said to be an expression of the quality of the orgasm. Others would argue that all orgasms are quality. During the peak of orgasm, usually lasting less than 30 seconds, heart rates may reach 160-180 beats per seconds, and breathing rates may exceed 40 per minute.

The Fourth Stage – Resolution

What is the definition of eternity? A comedian would say that it is the time between orgasm and leaving your partner's apartment on a less than perfect date. Others might answer that it is the time it takes for a man to regain the ability to experience a successful erection and second orgasm. However, all good things must come to an end and the intense blood flow to the genitals and the rest of the body following orgasm rapidly subsides. Peace has returned to the pelvic organs.

The Fifth Stage Which is The First Stage: Sexual Desire

If you thought sex was confusing and at times frustrating, you are right. Indeed, the fifth stage of the physiology of sex actually occurs before the first stage and was added on after the publication of the Masters and Johnson research. Kaplan and Lief were the first to discuss the fact that 30% of patients seen in sexual consultancy complained of a lack of desire. There may be many reasons desire is absent including mental and environmental issues. Desire is determined in part by attraction to the partner and deeper rooted fears, prior rejection and feelings of guilt. The ideal state for successful and pleasing sex is a similar level of desire between the two partners (occurring every 1012 years by astrological calculations). Sexual desire may also be affected by medications and medical conditions like heart disease and depression. Hormonal imbalances of the thyroid, adrenal glands, hypothalamus and sexual organs may be to blame.

One way to possibly enhance sexual desire is to ditch meat so you smell better. Yes, you read that right. There is science that indicates that non-meat eaters do smell better and therefore are more attractive. Seriously? Seventeen male volunteers ate a diet of meat for 2 weeks and one without meat for the same period (https://www.ncbi.nlm.nih.gov/pubmed/16891352). During the study, odor samples from the armpits of these men were collected and judged by 30 women as to the attractiveness of the smell! During the two weeks without meat, women judged the men's odors as more attractive, more pleasant, and less intense. You might meet the one that raises your sexual interest if you stop eating meat.

Now that you understand far more about forks, knives and fornication than you probably did before, let's turn to the role of plants and herbs in your pants.

CHAPTER 5

Plants and Herbs
in Your Pants

You exercise, you eat kale salads, watermelon, pine nuts, and arugula smoothies and you still are hungering for more sexual prowess, duration, and bravado. Where do you turn to if you shun prescription drugs like Viagra and the like (not to mention the price tag for one of these pills)? You turn to herbs because there is plenty of data and experience that putting plants in your pants can take your sexual fire even higher. So many of my patients have found that single herbs and "adaptogens" or combinations of groups of sexually stimulating and supportive plant based substances can raise their interest and success in the carnal arts. Let's look at some of the most useful plant based preparations that might just take your Vegan Sex to a higher plane (or in an airplane).

1. Maca

Maca is formally known as Lepidium Meyenii and grows in the Andes of Peru. It is grown predominantly for the reported value of its root that powered the Incan empire and its warriors. The powder of the root is considered safe to eat and contains glucosinolates similar to cruciferous vegetables like broccoli. Maca has been reported in testimonials to increase sexual performance in both men and women as well as symptoms of menopause in women. It is widely available in powder forms and capsules and in combination preparations. There are many scientific references for maca root including at least some actual scientific support that it enhances sexual performance (https://www.ncbi.nlm.nih.gov/pubmed/19260845).

2. Tribulus

Tribulus is an extract of an herb called Tribulus terrestris that contains many active agents including steroidal saponins, sterols and other compounds. Tribulus compounds together to reportedly help support normal reproductive function in men and women, help support normal hormone production in men and women promote vitality and stamina, support physical endurance, and to promote an overall feeling of well-being and sexual prowess. In a rare study of sexual responsiveness in women, tribulus was compared to placebo and increased the sexual interest of women with previously low interest (https://www.ncbi.nlm.nih.gov/pubmed/24773615). This has led some medical experts requesting that tribulus be added to drinking water (I am that expert).

3. Epimedium

Epimedium is a plant that comes from the botanical family 'Berberidaceae and derives mainly from China. As an aphrodisiac, it is better known as "horny goat weed".

The epimedium plant contains certain chemical compounds known as flavonoids that have antioxidant properties and plant based phytoestrogens that are weak like soy. This phytoestrogen, known as epimedium icariin, increases our friend NO and may increase testosterone. The benefits may include a role as an extremely potent aphrodisiac. Epimedium has also been used in the treatment of erectile dysfunction. Finally, icariin may also improve the sexual health and performance of women due to the production of NO and subsequent improved blood flow of blood to the sexual organs, clitoris and vagina. In a study of men with ED, a compound containing epimedium was superior to placebo for better sexual performance (https://www.ncbi.nlm.nih.gov/pubmed/24146455).

4. Damiana

Damiana, also known as Turnera diffusa, is a low-growing plant with yellow flowers and fragrant leaves. It's native to the subtropical climates of southern Texas, Mexico, Central and South America, and the Caribbean. The leaves and stem are used to make a mild liquor. Damiana's has also been used as an herbal remedy for centuries. By the time the Spanish crossed the Atlantic, indigenous cultures had been using it for centuries as an aphrodisiac and bladder tonic. Damiana is said to help enhance sexual health. In a study of 108 women with low sexual interest, a preparation including damiana led to greater interest and satisfaction with sex compared to a placebo preparation (https://www.ncbi.nlm.nih.gov/pubmed/16959660). Another one I would rather see in the public water supply than fluoride.

5. L-Arginine

You learned of the role of L-arginine, an amino acid, as a precursor to NO production, particularly if the enzyme called eNOS (funny that it rhymes with penis) is functioning efficiently to pump out NO. This pathway won, in part, the Nobel Prize in Medicine in 1998. There are supplements that have L-arginine alone or in combinations that are enhance sexual responsiveness. L-arginine can be combined as L-arginine-HCl (hydrochloric acid) but a particularly interesting form is L-arginine alpha-ketoglutarate. When this from is broken down glutamine is released which may be beneficial for gut and brain health as a bonus to boner support. There are dozens of studies on L-arginine and sexual responsiveness with many supportive findings (https://www.ncbi.nlm.nih.gov/pubmed/21966881). There is a single study of patients who suffered a heart attack that did not favor using L-arginine in high doses, and I usually avoid it in patients with recent heart attack, but lower dose forms, particularly with L-arginine alpha-ketoglutarate, are likely fine. I especially like some combination L-arginine alpha-ketoglutarate supplements that combine dietary nitrates (red spinach) and polyphenols from grapes and apples that boost the function of eNOS and provide a triple powered support for NO production and sexual performance.

6. Bergamot

Bergamot is citrus that looks like a lemon and grows on a tree only in the region of Southern Italy called Calabria, very close to Sicily. The fruit pulp has a unique combination of flavonoid chemicals like naringin, bruteridin, and melitidin. These natural compounds block the same enzyme that statin medications like Lipitor block without the concern over side effects. Bergamot has also been shown to lower blood sugar, lower inflammation, improve blood vessel activity, and activate the AMPK system similar to a popular diabetic drug called metformin.

Does bergamot work in patients? The science says yes and my experience does too. In a recent trial in 77 patients with high cholesterol, subjects were treated with a statin medication alone or combined with bergamot. The combination therapy produced the lowest LDL cholesterol and the highest HDL cholesterol. In addition, measures of damage to blood vessels by oxidation were the lowest with when bergamot was added. In other studies, the beneficial effects of bergamot on blood sugar levels and body weight were demonstrated. In other studies bergamot can help clear non-alcoholic fatty liver disease and a condition known as the metabolic syndrome. But what about sex?

When bergamot is combined with other herbal preparations, it has been shown to reverse ED in men with diabetes mellitus (http://www.sciencedirect.com/science/article/pii/S2213434415300256). This may be in part by supporting healthy blood sugar, blood pressure, and blood cholesterol. It may also be due to its powerful antioxidant properties that can improve endothelial function. It can be safely used in women too and is essentially free of side effects. It is as good as it sounds and is a supplement I take daily just for the sexual fun of it!

7. Magic Velvet Bean

Yes, there is a sexual enhancing herb called Magic Velvet Bean, more likely to be the name of a dancer at a club near an airport. This herb has been used for sexual support, infertility and nervous disorders and is also known by its chemical name mucuna pruriens of the Fabaceae family (no relationship to Fabio). It derives from ancient Indian Aryuvedic sources and is a powerful antioxidant that favors healthy arteries. Extracts of the seeds and leaves are available in various combination preparations to support successful sexual outcomes. There are reports of its activity in darkening hair and improving measures of Parkinson's disease. In the arena of sexual success, more data is available for Magic Velvet Bean improving sperm motility and potentially fertility (something you may be interested in or perhaps the quite the opposite). Clearly, this aryuvedic herb has activity on matters of sex (https://www.ncbi.nlm.nih.gov/pubmed/22499723).

8. Eurycoma Longifolia (Tongkat Ali)

This flowering plant with the two names above grows in Indonesia, Malaysia and Vietnam. It is used for medicinal purposes in those regions. The root of the plant can be boiled in water, and the water is consumed as a health tonic and as an aphrodisiac. In some cultures, the leaves can also be used as a source of bio active compounds.

In Western societies, E. longifolia is generally known as an aphrodisiac. Does it really work? There have a number of scientific research studies in humans carried out on E. longifolia towards analyzing its benefits. In a review of the medical literature published between 2000 and 2014, 11 studies of high quality were identified. In those studies, 7 of the 11 found strong associations between using this supplement and improved sexual health and performance (https://www.ncbi.nlm.nih.gov/pubmed/28259255).

In another evaluation of studies on E. Longifolia on erectile function, 2 studies involving 139 subjects were reported. Significant improvement in measures of erectile performance were measured particularly in those with the poorest performance on entry to the study (https://www.ncbi.nlm.nih. gov/pubmed/26365449). This herb is known to have antioxidant and anti-inflammatory actions that likely improve ED and lead to enhanced sexual performance.

Overall, the best route to preserve and enhance sexual performance is to lead a lifestyle most favorable to artery health. This would include absence of smoking, regular exercise, maintaining normal blood pressure, blood sugar, blood cholesterol, and achieving an ideal body weight. The best route to achieve these parameters is a whole food plant-based diet. For some that already have endothelial dysfunction leading to sexual impairment, the range of herbs outlined above alone or in combinations may support and enhance successful sexual activities. At the end of the day, plants can rock your sexual health whether eaten whole, or if needed, added as supplemental dried herbal preparations. Indeed, vegan sex is the best sex, the most sustained sex, and the healthiest sex. It may also be the kinkiest sex in a web based survey of habits of vegetarians versus non-vegetarians (https://theblog.okcupid. com/10-charts-about-sex-47e30d9716b0).

CHAPTER 6

The Epiphany: Mind-blowing Differences Between Vegan and Non-Vegan Sex
Gaining and Losing Love as a Vegan

As you might expect in the roller coaster of love, finding a soulmate who is also vegan is, I hate to say it, but yes–the vegan evangelism label I endured from a now ex husband–it was true.

I take ownership of the soapbox. When you find a partner on the soapbox with you, sharing the same religion, drinking the same kool-aid-- it's love at first and last sight--and everything in-between. To have the vegan connection is like no other, I believe. It takes you to the mountaintop like nothing else ever will. But the more passionately we love, the harder we fall. You would think that the vegan connection, once cemented, is forever. Until death do us part, or somewhere along that continuum. Warning: the pain of breaking up with someone who is vegan, combined with all the other stuff that melds a solid relationship is also like no other.

Spoiler alert: being vegan doesn't make you a whole person. It doesn't protect against the atrocities and damage that may have occurred in early or later life which may be problematic in building a long-term relationship. Just because your partner is vegan, you are not guaranteed a life of bliss, ideal companionship and wild and crazy love in and out of bed. The long-term success of a relationship is still determined by the massive glue that holds any successful relationship together: trust, respect, deep commitment to pleasing and honoring the other, fun, laughter, and putting the needs of the other before oneself. Veganism is but one large piece of a huge puzzle. Sometimes, it is easier to start a relationship with someone who isn't vegan, but who is open to the information and then connects the dots in a big way. The gratitude someone feels when they have improved their health as the result of your example and information is one of the most rewarding feelings you can ever experience. There is no finer paycheck.

You would think that the very definition of veganism automatically makes a person more loving, compassionate, giving, feeling and caring. If someone cares enough about helping animals, then it would seem logical that they would treat humans with equal compassion. Sometimes yes. Sometimes no. Humans are complex. A person with unhealed childhood or even adult wounds may consciously or unconsciously use animals for consolation in failed relationships. Animal causes may serve as their safe haven and respite. They may prefer the protection and unconditional love animals give over the risky behavior we humans offer, along with a huge risk of being hurt. Animals often offer the illusion or the reality of safe haven from a cruel and unkind world. No arguing that it is serving a higher good. Whatever works for the animals, right? They don't care as long as we care. They don't have time for us to figure ourselves out.

For me, the hardest thing to let go in my vegan pursuit and dreams was the deep and hard admission that it was not a guarantee. Just like some of my running friends believe that their running is their insurance policy that allows them to chow down on donuts, butter and all things meat and dairy after a long training run or race, vegan relationships are as varied as the food on our plates. It is not a guarantee of a match made in heaven, as much as it might seem to be. In fact, they can be every bit as crazy as relationships with omnis. Some of my women friends argue that some of their worst relationships were with vegans. Do we become vegan because of some hurt we had early in life which made us more sensitive to the needs and abuses of animals? Is being kind and compassionate toward animals a way of healing the hurts of childhood and later in life? Is kindness toward animals a replacement for quality therapy that might have healed those deep wounds better than taking care of animals? As one of my fav running shirts says, "Running is cheaper than therapy." Is loving animals a replacement for therapy? I simply pose the questions. Only you can answer them.

Features and Benefits of Vegan Partners: Pro and Con

Like the endorphins of running, there is nothing like a vegan high. I can remember it as if it were yesterday. I was in a restaurant with my vegan love. The waitress saw his shirt and began peppering him with questions about what it was like to be vegan. Without missing a beat, he answered a dozen questions citing research, experience and loving the moment of outreach, whenever it shows up. I remember an almost out of body experience watching us all at the table. I felt so proud, happy and grateful that I could relish and take in the moment. I was proud of him, proud of us and so happy to be there. I have never felt so in sync with anyone. Was it the rose-colored glasses of blinding, irrational love? Was it that he was just so good in bed that I couldn't imagine another partner as giving, considerate and OK, I'll just say it, hard and long-lasting?

When the relationship crashed and burned, I could not at all understand why. How could he let it go? Did he not know how good he had it? Or was every vegan babe as good as me, whatever that could possibly mean on a physical, intellectual and emotional level? How could anyone be as good as me, I would egotistically ask myself, and even him once? After seeing some the posts and videos from one of my "competitors," I thought, OK, if that's the kind of self-serving bimbette he wants, buh-bye now.

What a difference time can make. Fast forward a year. Another vegan love did exactly the same thing: totally quoting line and verse from some vegan bible to a waitress at her first questions. Over time, I would encourage him to attend with me the largest vegan events of the year such as Healthfest or North American Vegetarian Summerfest. He would say, "No dear, I'd rather learn it all from you." I got it. We all want someone to be our clipping service, wading through the avalanches of information online and off.

The coolest thing about this experience is that my love was not vegan the year before. He started his journey because of me. And in the beautiful raw food restaurant, when a couple at the nearby table started peppering him with questions, these random strangers had no hesitation asking him about veganism changed his life. He responded to every question and went "there" saying how he could feel the change and improved blood flow in his lungs and sexual organs. Another couple at nearby table was all ears too.

But a year before, when I was submerged by the old drama with the old love, all I can say is I'm sure glad I didn't grow up with Facebook. Having the photos, the videos and the lovey-dovey chit-chats of an ex with their new lover or rekindled ex-lover probably would have made me suicidal or homicidal in my youth. In my more mature years, at least I have the strength to unfriend or just turn off the computer and go for a run.

On a rational level I could justify our breakup, because he had his reasons. And well, reasons are reasons with guys. I've read that a broken heart is actually a very physical phenomenon. It can take some time, years even, to get over it. Like a physical wound, emotional wounds can go deep. A vegan diet doesn't give you thick skin or a heart or coat of armour. You are fairly warned that a vegan partner is no guarantee against heartbreak.

If anything, it can be as rugged as anything you'll experience. And maybe more so, because you thought your mutual veganism, shared beliefs, values and common goals made a bond stronger than Super Glue soulmates in the truest form.

Veganism is often the cement that wraps around all the other components of a solid relationship. The partnerships that do succeed are unlike no other because they have that extra component of serving a higher good, the cause, being on the same side of the good fight, the right side of history. There are a number of vegan "partnerships" that glow like no other relationships or marriages. If you know any of these couples, some on the national lecture circuit, perhaps you've had the opportunity to witness their chemistry. The spark between them when they talk is like a thousand suns of hopeful light.

But for those who don't have it so lucky and see their relationships crumble, it is devastating. Like runners who think they have an insurance policy against eating burgers, bacon and all things unhealthy, vegans sometimes think that loving another vegan means they'll fly high forever. Not so fast, Sherlock. Not long after my heartbreak, fortunately, I found that a new friend was receptive to the vegan message due to his health problems. We began dating and eventually, he shared with me that he had a prescription for Viagra. He told me that he had not had sex in a very long time. Decades, in fact. He tried it for a couple times during our sexual encounters, but then, as you might expect, he no longer needed it. Not at all. Never looked back. This my friends, can be your story too.

My experiences put in stark contrast the difference between vegan men and non vegan men. As an investigative reporter, I often got asked and still do, "What are the main qualities that make a good investigative reporter?" Without missing a beat, I always answer, an insatiable curiosity and a huge sense of righteous indignation that fires up the brain at the slightest injustice. With my first vegan sexual encounter, and then even more with my second, the questions lit up my brain like a million firecrackers. Why is there such a difference? What are the differences, emotionally and physically? If all men knew how much better it was, physically and emotionally, but especially physically, wouldn't we have a lot more vegans in the world? And the loudest, angriest question of all: "Why didn't my doctor tell me this?" I hope you ask yourself these questions and many more too.

The Physical Differences Between Vegan and Omni Sex

As I've hinted at earlier, there are incredibly distinct differences between vegan and non-vegan sex. I recently mentioned to a non-vegan that I was writing this book. She angrily flew off at me like nobody ever had saying, "There are so many causes of ED, you can't say that diet causes it!" Turns out, her husband had prostate cancer, and she initially thought that I was suggesting that a plant-based diet would reverse the damage cancer and its treatment had done to their sex life.

When I explained that a vegan diet could prevent ED in the first place, well before a cancer diagnosis, she still didn't want to go there. The emotional charge of the topic alone, aside from all the research and facts tied into the causes and prevention on ED are so volatile, it is hard for people affected by the related conditions and diseases to even listen to the "other" side.

For some, it's too little too late. My best friend who died of breast cancer asked late in her diagnosis about a plant-based diet. For her, it seemed to help a little bit. But it was too late. She never saw her youngest child make it to high school. This is not to say a vegan diet could have prevented her breast cancer. It is not a 100% guarantee. Vegans do get cancer. But not nearly the rate that the meat-eating, high-fat devouring populations do. The lifetime of work by Dr. Neal Barnard and his nonprofit, Physicians Committee for Responsible Medicine, is based on his research and that of others which gave birth to the Cancer Project nonprofit. The Cancer Project trained cooking instructors like me who in turn then tried to help people how to eat a healthful vegan

VEGAN SEX

diet with free or almost free cooking classes. I was honored to train and teach those classes for six years and saw all kinds of "spontaneous remissions" with students reversing many conditions and coming off medications for diabetes, heart disease and high blood pressure. No commercials for that on TV. No money in broccoli.

There has been and will probably always continue to be as long as the meat and dairy industries have their powerful influence in and on Washington, a huge campaign by special interests to discredit the work of the courageous hero vegan doctors. These doctors chose decades ago to protest conventional wisdom by practicing preventative medicine and writing books that would speak from their hearts and their own very real experience in witnessing blue zones and longevities that were centered in cultures around the world that were surprise, surprise, plant-based.

The Vegan Edge: Foreplay

We live in a slam-bam thank-you ma'am gotta have it now sexual revolution. But if an erection can last for hours, what's the rush? Your man can take his time caressing your every nook and cranny, leaving no place untouched. There is nothing quite like an erect penis teasing nerve endings in the most sensitive perimeter of the vaginal opening. After 30 or 60 minutes of that, you might be begging your man to please enter. Or if you're the man, you might be dreaming up or finding distractions to keep from entering your woman before she is begging and clamoring for it. Ah...first world vegan problems. Bring it!

Ejaculation

Since I can only write this from my personal experience, which is a non-medical, non-clinical perspective, my experience is that ejaculation from a vegan penis is way, WAY more sensual and powerful than from an omni. Because the guy can last a long, long time, the race to the finish line can take a long time too. The act of ejaculation or orgasm for the woman builds more slowly, pretty much regardless of the age. For the woman, that means you can feel the blood swelling inside the penis as semen builds in his testicles, and inside you. It is almost like you have this imaginary countdown clock. You can really feel when your man is about to come. And that leads us to the next plateau:

Simultaneous Orgasms

Because both partners are so in tune with each other on the deepest internal physical experience, it is, dare I say, almost easy to have simultaneous orgasms. Often, it is the woman who has more control over when she attains an orgasm. But if she gets clear signals from her man, and I don't mean only verbal cues of heavy breathing, there is no question of when her man is about to explode inside her. She can definitely feel the pulsating penis growing and throbbing within her. Pardon the steamy, almost pornographic language. But when you've had this experience, especially when you thought previously you were way over the hill, that sex was a thing of the past and not in your future, your mind is forever blown. You become a believer.

Men who have not had sex in an eternity, and we're even including masterbation in this category, those who really didn't think it could ever happen again, are passionate vegans for the rest of their lives. They are living testimonials of just how powerful a vegan diet can be. Even at the age of 70 or beyond, previously dead sex--we're talking dead for decades--can come back like a roaring fire engine.

Vegan Virgin: The Saga of Nick

I personally experienced this in a rather comical way. Gulp. This may be the most personal and intimate part of my sexuality that I will share. All for the cause, of course. All for the animals. Including human ones. Here goes.

I had not had intercourse in decades. That's right. Decades. I had hung in there with my ex, actually several exes, who had ED. The only way one of them could have an orgasm was through masterbation or oral sex. First of all, he was so obese that he could not get on top of me without my feeling like my stomach and lungs were about to be crushed. His belly was so distended that my getting on top was impossible as well. When our relationship crumbled, I had an opportunity with a guy I'll call Nick that I thought might result in intercourse. I went to my doctor to get a baseline of STD tests to show I was clean.

I had been experiencing back pain and the doctor thought the pain might be related to a prolapsing uterus, which can be common in premenopausal or menopausal women, or even runners like myself. Uterine muscles stretched from pregnancy, childbirth and gravity relax to the point where it can be seen in the vagina or worse, lower right out of the vagina. The doctor referred me to a rather interesting physical therapist he thought might be able to help. I had no idea what was about to happen.

The therapist specialized in helping women strengthen their pelvic floors or in simple language, not give birth to their uteruses. She also worked with men as well. And so began one of the most unusual "evaluations" I had ever had. Keep in mind, as a runner for 35 years, I had seen my share of traditional physical therapists who do traditional evaluations of feet, knees, hips and other appendages. But this PT did an internal probe of my innards like no other therapist. She measured the degree of prolapse and atrophy of various muscles of the vaginal wall. Her prescription? A dildo. In fact, after taking measurements, she said she would go with a co-worker to purchase one at the nearby X-rated adult toy store. What? A health care professional whose job included buying dildos for patients? And health insurance paid for it?

A week later, at the next appointment, she came back with a long, white, slender, soft silicone covered vibrating dildo. Her instructions, "This is not necessarily to get you to the point of climaxing. The goal is for your to have the dildo act as a massage of your muscles that have atrophied from not having intercourse all these years. When the muscles tighten, your uterus won't feel like it's about to fall out. The dildo will help stimulate the nerves and encourage blood flow. It's the old use it or lose it in play here." It all sounded very clinical to me. I don't know if it really worked, but during the time period I kept my appointments, I told her that I had an opportunity to have sex that might result in intercourse with a new partner.

She immediately had a very concerned and serious look on her face. "You're going to need lubricants because it will be very painful. Your vaginal walls have thinned and you're not as flexible as you used to be in that part of your body. You'll need to keep doing your 100 slow and fast kegels twice a day."

I stocked up on three different kinds of lubricants, making sure they were vegan, and if possible, organic. Of course. When I went to Nick's house where the "activity" was to occur, I secretly slid the lubricants under my pillow. But lo and behold, as the evening unfolded, in fact as the entire week of love-making unfolded, I didn't need a single one of the damn lubricants. Nope. Not a one. I returned a couple of them to the pharmacy and got my money back. As I should have. I left one of them under the pillow as a surprise for Nick, and a reminder of how far, forgive the pun, I had come.

I went back to the physical therapist, not because I needed to, but just to tell her that she was dead wrong. I gushed about how my partner glided in and out of me like a well vegan-buttered cucumber. My juices gushed and flowed for hours, I gushed. Her response when I bragged that I didn't need the recommended artificial lubricants, "Oh, that's just the newness of the relationship. This too will fade."

Spoiler alert mainstream health care professionals: It didn't fade. Our relationship prevailed for more than a year, and there were never any sexual problems. We both professed undying friendship because he couldn't use the "R" (relationship) or "L" (love) words. We both spoke of how our mutual passion for veganism carried well into bedroom passion. We would both say to each other that it was the best sex each of us had ever had, whatever that meant. For me, it meant a deep caring and sharing, a mutuality that resulted in frequent orgasms for both of us, and often, coming at the same time, or close to it. For those in their 60's and beyond, I think that's pretty remarkable and amazing. And, I'm guessing, friggen rare. I rarely had simultaneous orgasms except in my twenties.

I have no idea if for Nick, it really was the best sex of his life. I knew that being the stud he was and is, my escapade with him didn't begin or end with me. As one of my male friends who lent me a crying shoulder when this passion fizzled, said, "Aw c'mon, the guy probably doesn't have but a decade or two, maybe three, if he's lucky to live. He should have as much fun as he can." Ah...the male mind.

Unbeknownst to me at the time when we met, Nick was not at all available to be in a relationship with anyone. He gave me a long list of women he felt "confused" about where he was going in those relationships. Part of my reason for getting sucked into the harem I almost mocked during the first conversation Nick and I ever had, was quite frankly, I hadn't had intercourse or any remotely kind of romantic sex in decades. What little I had, felt purely functional to keep the parts in good working order, and usually the parts weren't mine. In other words, my partner was so focused on his own sexual dysfunction, I was focused on doing what I could to alleviate that. I had shoved sexual pleasure and satisfaction for myself into a shoebox on a shelf dismissing it as "not important." In short, I was lonely. Yeah, even PETA's Sexiest Vegan over 50 got lonely.

Another guy I knew told me on our first date that he told every woman he dated that he had "commitment phobia." He almost seemed proud of it. At least I was clear from the get-go where he stood. Or got laid. But things were murky with Nick. The first time I met him, he too, listed the long entourage of women who were after him in the past year. I joked with him about his harem. It wasn't a harem, he said. Of course it is, I argued cheerfully and expressed confidence that he was a bright boy and would figure it all out, or just enjoy the ride.

The dilemma of the hotly pursued, vegan male. Nick fit the role to a "T." Of course, hot mama that I thought I was, modesty aside, like most women, yes, I thought if anyone could wow this challenge, that would be me. One of many articles written about me over my TV career was headlined, "Consumer Reporter Loves a Challenge." Yup. My mama always told me, "You can't change the world." "Watch me try," I would silently vow. Still trying to prove her wrong apparently, bless her loving good soul. She was only trying to spare her babies a little pain.

But I did think I could break the wall down, even though I talked a good "friends with benefits" lie. In the end, the lie was to myself. I thought I could hack it. I was so sex starved that I was content and gave healthy doses to both of us the mantra, "Let's just live in the moment." I truly believed we were. I believed that if it all ended tomorrow, I would be fine. I would have the sweet memories of the best sex of my life, and that was that. Oh, that women could borrow a little of the male "I must move on now" mentality.

I thought I had coated my heart in stainless steel. If you can do that, it is all about just being in the moment. If I had a nickel for every time I uttered that phrase as an affirmation for myself and a directive to Nick so that he could stop stressing about where our non-relationship was or wasn't going, I could make a hefty donation to PETA.

But alas, I would ultimately lose the battle to the stiff competition. Problem was, I really didn't need anything. I wasn't needy other than a little love, appreciation and respect. I didn't need money or attention to tend to a crazy-making drama meltdown. Nick seemed to thrive, as many men do, in a caretaker role. The more rescuing and help a woman needed, the crazier she was, by his own descriptions, the more he was at her side. The damsel in distress modality is alive and well.

I definitely had my own identity. But as I learned in my TV career, while this sounds a bit old school, it is often hard for men to cope with strong women.

The main observation in 20/20 hindsight vision is my biggest "flaw" was that I was available. And I don't play games. Nick definitely seemed most connected and engaged with women who weren't available--either physically, living far away, or emotionally so wrapped up in their own drama that he loved to rush in and try to be the rescuer. Some men really thrive in that role. By picking women who were about as unavailable as he was, there was no chance any of those relationships would seriously go anywhere. Nick had a long list of complaints about each woman, and why she could never be stable, confident or smart enough to be his soulmate. I had this aced, or so I thought. But I don't play games well, and my life has since gone on a much healthier trajectory. As was predicted, we all have our transition relationships.

Nick and I remain distant, occasional friends, as difficult and painful as that has been for me. There have been times, in our social media world, where I want to unfriend and disconnect. I really don't like seeing his thumbnail face pop up first in my Messenger favorites. I suppose Facebook algorithms will change that eventually one day. Yet I don't pull the plug. My self-doubts kick in chiding my inner voices, "Whatsamatter with you? You don't need him. He treated you badly. And he's treated others the same way. Dump the guy."

Yet, what inspired me in his posts ages ago, still does. It is the dedication to the cause, and the amount of time and thoughtfulness that attracted me in the first place that still keeps me connected and at the least, interested in what he is thinking and writing. That's what makes it so hard to disconnect, I rationalize. And that's the rub for us vegans. We make exceptions for our partners because they are vegan. We give them a pass, or many passes because we know how hard it is to find a vegan partner.

One time I was almost about to delete his Facebook friendship when I thought, I'll copy all of our messages from Messenger, just in case those disappear. Facebook had recently installed a function where you could delete individual messages. As I scrolled back a year and half through the mangroves of passion, despair and brilliance, I cried one last time, shaking my head in disbelief. How could he have lied? How could he have said all that stuff and reneged? It was truly, his loss. I'd like to believe that he had no clue what he was losing. But deep down, he knew.

He truly didn't deserve me, I self-talked. Rarely to we get to such points in our lives where we feel so deeply hurt. But even if your love is a superstar vegan, if he doesn't love you for exactly who you are, it is definitely time to move on. One of these days, I may get the courage to unfriend him on Facebook. Part of me wants to try it just to see if he'd even notice, because he is so wrapped up in his own drama that it could be months, years or maybe never before realized the breakup was official on social media. However, I would never really know if he noticed unless he messaged, which is most unlikely. Such first world problems in middle school drama. It all seems so trivial when you consider how much work needs to be done to save the planet and our own lives. Yet, at the time, it is deep pain when you experience it.

One of my friends shared with me some great advice and a beautiful passage she sent to break up with a boyfriend who had ripped her heart out too. It was so gracious and full of love and compassion that only a vegan on the verge of heartbreak would have to offer. She was still primarily thinking of the other instead of her painful suffering.

"So, here's some wisdom I have gained that I can share:

1. I send a golden cord of light from my heart to the person that I am having difficulty with. With my boyfriend, I would send and think, 'I send you pure love and light from my heart to yours. For whatever you need. Wholeness in all ways possible.' It definitely changed me and I felt that it made my communication easier and from a place of love (rather than fear/ ego).

2. I acknowledge fully: this or something better, for the greatest good of all involved. (And I know that ALL includes both me and him). So, I can love him fully and be willing to walk away if we don't share a common vision. As I am sure you know, and I am just *reminding* you ;), without a common vision, there can be no sustainable relationship.

3.   I reminded myself that if this relationship was for my highest and best, then I didn't need to do anything but be most my loving, highest and best self. If it was a good relationship, it would move further into my life. And if it was not good for me, then it would move out of my life.

4.   Finally, and most importantly, I remembered that the future is based on the NOW. If the now isn't good, the future won't be. And at that time in that NOW, it wasn't good. I even told my boyfriend, 'The future is based on the now. And I want to create a good now. If you're not available, we need to stop this. I send you love, light and an abundance of all good things in all dimensions of time - and I release you for whatever pathway you need to take.'

Of course, my heart was breaking when I did that. But I knew I had to do that.

All we can ever do is be clear with who we are and the vision we would like to create. We can't bring someone else on board or get them to have our vision. We can hold a space with love and allow what will be - that person moving further in or slowly out."

As I read point 4 above, the "Dear John" text that my friend sent to her boyfriend and recommended that I do the same, I just couldn't. I love and respect her dearly for being able to do that. But I just couldn't go there. Instead, I never officially ended our relationship on my end. He ended it on his end long ago. I let it, the non-relationship dangle and twist in the wind. It is so hard to create closure and wish someone good fortune when they've emptied your bank of stored, treasured and precious feelings of love. I wasn't up to the "have a wonderful life" parting line. Although I have read and re-read what my friend wrote above many times just to console myself. Call me cranky and bitter. But charitable at the end of a relationship is the one time in life I feel a little stingy and protective of my feelings.

Another friend who had observed our non-relationship relationship in action as best anyone can from afar recommended sending this, which I did not:

"I love you, I want to share a life with you but you're clearly not ready so I'm letting you go. If you want me, you're going to have to prove it. But I'm not waiting around anymore waiting for your proof. In the meantime, I'm going on with my life."

Further she advised, "Take a week to weep and be with good friends then allow yourself to get taken out, treated well and make sure that SOB sees it. Do NOT apologize for shit!!!!

Remember your self worth. Remember he should be begging you to be with him.

You're both adults except he's not stepping up to the plate. I hate childish men, mama's boys. Grow the fuck up man! Now that I got that out of my system, lol."

I tried to defend the guy with the problems from his early childhood, but my best bud would not have any of that. I texted:

"I try to be compassionate and understanding of how that may affect him ways he's not aware. But you're right. thanks!!!"

"Oh boo hoo, he's how old now?"

"Damn too few vegan men in the world."

I did not say any of that either to my ex, but I have read it from time to time, and it has helped me refocus on why I began this journey in the first place. That one line in particular rang so true, as I hope it does for you, male or female, "he should be begging me to be with him."

How Low Can You Go?

In the course of my journey, and in part because I was starting to write this book, I began researching the male brain and behavior in earnest. Gulp. Big confession. I spent hundreds of dollars on the programs that the loneliest of the loneliest purchase. These sites sure prey on our insatiable desire to be loved, at almost any cost. "BeIrresistable.com." "Text Your Ex Back." "AddictHim.com." There was even one memorable e-book, "Why Men Always Lie." I have no recollection of what those reasons were, and I am sure they were excellent rationalizations for why men lie, other than they just do. So don't take it personally, if you're a guy reading this.

The many ClickBank sites like these go and on, laughing all the way to the real bank. Fess up. Who among you feels my pain and has visited and, oh dear, invested hard earned money on these one liners or 20 minute videos you can't stop watching that prey on the lonely? Filled with promises and deep secrets of how their methods can make your man proposing marriage in just hours, the promise of at least getting the most resistant guy back in your arms is too good to pass up.

The good news? These sites all have money back guarantees. If you're not happy, they'll gladly refund your $47, $97 or whatever amount you forked over during the multiple upsell pages that kept hounding you and pounding different ways to entice a guy. Usually the refund is granted, no questions asked. One time I called my credit card company when a charge was not credited. When the credit card company heard that I was disputing a ClickBank charge, the operator let out a loud sigh of exasperation. "Want me to put a freeze on your card so they can't charge those secret monthly charges you didn't realize you'd signed up for? Or we can ban them completely from your card so even if you try to order from them again, you can't. They have so many complaints." Wait...did I just get scolded for not being able to manage my loneliness dollars? So be it. Ban me and my credit cards from these companies who profit on the lonely. So there.

As if any of these programs would help me or anyone. But maybe they do. Maybe they at least help some of us to feel we are not the only ones going through this kind of pain. However, I did learn a few things and discovered patterns of male behavior after hearing the same information among the different ebooks and hardcover books. Among them, men do think often about women and sex, like every 7 seconds or 7 minutes, whichever statistic you want to believe. The thought process is tied more to their anatomy, and not their brains. Some have described it bluntly, men think with their penis. They are hardwired to go after their women, in a big way. Playing hard to get is not a game, but it is what women often do before they decide who will be their partner. That game of courtship brings out the creativity and romanticism in both sexes. In the process, men usually resort to physical activity to try to please their partners. He will build. He will buy flowers. He will rearrange or buy furniture to feather the nest. He will tear out the landscaping, weed like there's no tomorrow and start all over in landscape design. He will text photos of it to prove his undying love, in case you are not there to witness it. He will respond to brief graphic images of scantily clad and nude photos that appeal to his basic instincts. Or as one book, "Everyday Dad" describes it, "a man's brain has two lobes: the 'Oh yeah baby I'm thinking about sex' lobe which takes up 88% of the brain, and 'Future Sites of Dreams' about supermodels takes up 10%, and and the 'Everything Else' takes up 2%. The broadband connection in women's brains allows them to multi-task. In a man's brain...we can only focus on one task at a time, and if we are interrupted while we are working on the task, our brain experiences a fatal error." So glad that was written by a guy taking ownership. Yeah, baby!

I remember one time, probably when Nick and I were the closest emotionally, he really couldn't handle it. I could just sense it. We spent a couple of days weeding and gardening until the place looked like something out of Better Homes and Gardens. I don't think I ever worked so hard and sweated so much, even in a Florida marathon. He continued to perfect his landscaping, bushwhacking and climbed trees like a monkey to clip branches. I got nervous, sweaty palms just watching his acrobatic feats. But I've seen more than one almost 70-something man climb trees with masterful agility and without fear--all perhaps to impress their women.

Nick, like so many halfway decent and kind men, vegan or not, are in high demand. For them, it is often a confusing and long road. When I think of all the women I know who have thrown themselves at him, it's no wonder men who are hotly pursued are confused. In one conversation, they may tell you that they're looking for a soulmate, and you're as darn close as anybody has come in the last half century. But when the knocking at the door resumes, as it always will, the walls break down, and the incredibly delicious man is available...for everyone else. Other women will tell you they've heard the same soulmate, best friend lines. Give him a beer or three, and he's all over reciprocating the advances of the most current assertive women. So it goes in the animal kingdom. What makes one man monogamous and another not? It is often hard to say. My short answer is that when a guy has a rugged breakup and is himself deeply hurt, he is more open to doing what it takes to please a woman in the next relationship. If a guy has always been the one doing the breaking up, interestingly, given that veganism is the definition of compassion in theory, he may not have the compassion to understand how awful being dumped can be. Walk a mile in my shoes, and you may want to appreciate the current relationship and not be so quick to move on to the next partner.

Others feel that this kind of relationship-aversion behavior is more indicative of someone who can't commit for all kinds of reasons and really has nothing to do with veganism. The belief is that veganism is just a characteristic like hair or eye color. It gets a little tricky here. Because the choice to eat and live vegan is voluntary, some believe that those who prey on the weak could use veganism as a cover to gain favor. They enter into a victim's life who has chosen veganism as a way to alleviate the pain and suffering experienced in an earlier traumatic event. That event could have been the victim, or even the perpetrator witnessing abuse to animals or humans, or both. Regardless of the cause, simply, the trauma always remains traumatic. The images, sounds and feelings may recede into the background, but they never disappear.

While some people are great at compartmentalizing and putting that trauma in a shoebox on a high shelf, others are walking wounded wearing heartaches and neediness on their sleeves. While I believe the sociopathic behavior to prey on victims who have chosen veganism as a cause for protection and escape is not common, it is definitely something to be aware of if you feel you may be in a vulnerable victim scenario. I recall that the president of a vegetarian club was ousted from his position when it became obvious that he was using his power to make sexually inappropriate advances to female club members. This can happen in any organization. But as vegans, we are under the microscope for our somewhat controversial beliefs anyway, and we may come under more intense scrutiny.

Odds are, if you choose to believe that people are basically good, intentions of your partners will be good too. You will have plenty of opportunities to see how actions will speak louder than words. In short, when you add "vegan" to a great man's bio, Katie bar the door. Lock the front door if you can. I don't mean that in a possessive sense. Or even that there is a way for you to control another. Of course there isn't. But to the extent a man is truly looking for a partner, only you can decide how much energy and time you want to devote to making that possibility a reality. I actually had a woman counsel me giving the sternest of lectures to never tell other women in real life or online that I was involved with a great guy, especially a vegan guy. She acted like some really aggressive women would be on the first flight to my front door. It's hard, but not impossible to stay mum about your personal life in today's world with social media and public events. Everyone anywhere can photograph instantly and share.

In our prime, my vegan guy said in the heat of a wonderful moment, "No matter what happens, let us promise ourselves we will never settle for anything less than what we have now." He said it almost as a closing argument to himself. In that moment, I knew we both had the best. At the time, I was sure I would never believe differently both from my perspective as well as his. In other words, I can't imagine that he could do better than me.

He had told me he liked me better than anyone so far. If you believe this was the best, why would you bail?

Personality disorders that affect men in particular in early childhood, the loss of a parent for example, can play out hugely in adulthood. Like a hurt puppy dog, a man can play the role of the abandoned child. He may look for love in all the right places and find it with women, no problem. He may attract quite a harem before all is said and done, claiming to like and love one more than the next. The littered trail of promised love and broken plans for a new kitchen, or even an entire home keep the victim enticed and interested. The dead giveaway is that no plans come to fruition. But when the next victim comes along, the player moves on.

It is important to really look at why an individual is vegan. On the surface, it may be for all the best reasons. But if veganism is used to cover or camouflage a deep hurt that has never been properly addressed, buyer beware. Be seriously aware.

Like veganism not being the insurance policy against all diseases, it is not the fail-safe, bullet-proof emotional armour for a man or woman. But especially for women who tend to be caring and compassionate in the vegan mold, they can also be an easy prey or victim to a man who is trying to avoid dealing with healing his early childhood hurts or adult traumas.

The demons that even vegans have are ones they must wrestle and fix themselves. Nobody can fix a bad childhood or a bad or even mediocre marriage. You can only give it your best shot. Knowing when to leave is part of the self-respect you owe yourself.

I knew that Nick's reminders that he wasn't available for a relationship was his way of saying, it ain't gonna last. So don't get your hopes up or panties in a wad. Did he use me? Yes, he admitted that he liked being seen with me. Ugh. Where are the men who ask questions about your day, or what they can do to help you each day? Fortunately, I would eventually find such a great vegan guy who eventually made me realize just how self-absorbed my perfect transitional vegan man was. I would swear months after Nick and I dissolved, that Taylor Swift song, "Wildest Dreams" had synchronistically been written for that moment:

"...Nothing lasts forever
But this is gonna take me down...
I can see the end as it begins
My one condition is
Say you'll remember me
Say you'll see me again even if it's just in your wildest dreams..."

We're all invested in our egos and beliefs about ourselves. If we believe positively in ourselves, as we are always told to do for healthy self-esteem, we can end up wondering and wandering into the depths, perhaps of despair, why some relationships don't work out. Sometimes you might hear, it's not you, it's me. While that can be true, sometimes it is just as simple as you could have been the best catch in the world, but your partner isn't ready and never will be, no matter what words come out of his or her mouth. Or perhaps you were too smart, too worldly, too passionate, too pressuring, even though you were sure you weren't, or too something that meant you were not meant to be. Or maybe you weren't too anything at all. Maybe it really was never about you to begin with.

The drama of social media allows anyone to "stalk" their competition. In today's world, it seems easy to say after checking out the competition's page, or worse, videos, you could easily drive yourself crazy saying things like, "he likes that dingbat over me?" Don't. Just don't. Move on. Be done. SO much easier said than done. But there are other vegans at the sanctuary. So hone those skills of compartmentalizing. Put the relationship in a shoebox and don't ever look at it again unless you must. I remember hearing that 50% of popular songs you hear on the radio or wherever your media source is, are about the beginning and honeymoon phase of a relationship, the other 50% is about the end or breakup. Pick a few. Roll up your car windows and sing and cry loudly. Let the healing begin. Love with a vegan can be a great soaring to the heavens, and equally so, a free fall into hell.

I still mourn over the loss of my relationship with Nick. But less and less as time heals all. That's the thing about loving as a vegan and loving someone who is vegan...because you have one more level of connectedness, the glue that holds you together is all that much harder to crack and break apart. The interesting thing is, it is the vegan connection that may keep you together as friends. No matter what else happens, I have always felt glad about that and perhaps always will. The more distance from the heat of the moment I give myself, the more I recognize that the relationship was flawed and pretty much all about him, his angst about his life's decisions, and more importantly, an acute lack of interest and real caring about my life. Being vegan can add rose-colored glasses which may cloud your judgement that otherwise would have been more rational and logical. Be ever vigilant.

I know this has been a long thread about the negative outcome of a vegan relationship. But I also hope it conveys the many positive attributes important to successful vegan relationships. Because we were both vegan, we had so much more in common. I know other vegan couples who say that too. I can't ever imagine being that much of a soulmate with someone ever again unless the vegan connection is solid. But therein lies the danger. Because Nick was vegan, that offered me an illusion of decency and courtesy that in retrospect, did not really exist. To a woman, a relationship with a vegan guy is so romantic. That can set the the stage for some pretty powerful delusions of your own.

Of course there is way more than just veganism to a long-lasting partnership...the qualities that ignite and continue to fuel the flames of emotional, intellectual and physical attraction. Yet, there is the self-pride that says, if your partner doesn't appreciate you enough to want to be with you, get over it. Life goes on.

You may argue with yourself, how will I really move on, or will I be stuck in the crevasse forever? You can stomp out a flame, but the coals and embers are more challenging. They ignite just when you think the last one is gone. Humans would probably be more than the messes they are if the old adage, "time heals all" didn't work. The brain and memory are fascinating manipulators of time, and with enough self-talk, you may be able to wiggle out of that seemingly endlessly deep canyon of heartache.

Friends will tell you you're way too cool and awesome to remain stuck on anyone who doesn't appreciate and/or love you for who you are, just the way you are. Ah...another concept so much easier said than done, isn't it? It can be easy to say, it was just a "transition" relationship. It got you out of one bad one, maybe even one with a carnivore who had no respect for your growing education and beliefs, and ejected you all that much closer to the next good relationship. Sounds a lot like the sales training I got on Wall Street...it takes 40 "nos" to get one yes. A phone slammed down in your ear is all that much closer to the next yes. Again, that it would be so easy.

I hope you understand the value of the public pity party. Many of us have been there, and it is so hard to pick up the pieces and move on. But we must do that and not wallow in toxic relationships. Having a strong, viable partnership can be important to those wanting to help animals, improve human health and save the environment. That is not to say you can't soldier on fighting the good fights without a partner. Indeed, more people live alone now than ever before. In the end, the decision to take a risk and go it alone rather than remaining in an unhealthy relationship rules the day.

After my rugged experience, it is understandable why some people find themselves deep into animal rights because they just give up in some or maybe all areas with people. It is so much easier to love a peaceful animal than a human being who talks back, argues, abuses, disrespects or doesn't appreciate. Animals love unconditionally. What is not to love about that? It is also way easier to focus on a cause higher than yourself to avoid staying too long at the pity party.

OK. Enough wallowing. On a positive note, on the flip side, and I'm guessing you may have had this happen too...a guy I went out with decided on the first date that I was "the one." Full of passion, energy and smart enough to be educated in veganism that might help his condition dujour, I met everything else on his checklist too. He blatantly told me fairly early on in our dating that he wanted to spend the rest of his life with me "to have fun and because having one partner minimizes risk of STD'S." Now there's a romantic line. Six months into the relationship, after watching "Forks Over Knives" and "Earthlings," he sent me two bacon jokes all in one day, including one that said, "Women are like bacon: They look good, smell good, taste good and slowly kill men." What part of the word "vegan" did he not understand? I became acutely aware that I sometimes don't have a sense of humor like some people think we vegans should. As the long, crazy Facebook thread erupts: Bacon! Whatever. Raising vegan men is so tough!

But people, including the male species can and do change. It is all dependent upon how much they want you which can be highly tied into their innate desire to please you. Milk that one for all it is worth, ladies. And men. Sometimes their desire to go vegan is all about winning your favor. But eventually, if the relationship lasts, they will take ownership of their journey, reasons and emotions. It's no longer so much about trying to please you as it is waking up one day and realizing, "Whoa, I feel better, I love better, and I love this food that I'm eating. And when I don't eat it, I feel like crap." All of a sudden, they understand what it really feels like to enjoy good health and the community of others who share the same values with the same fact set.

The interesting end to the Nick story is that in my next sexual encounter, once again, there was no problem lubricating. I did not experience any of those dire warnings of the painful, dryness scourge associated with a meat-eaters menopause as long as I drink plenty of water, and avoid alcohol and caffeine. I've been in that new relationship for almost a year, and again, the newness seems like it will never wear off. Piece of carrot cake. Take that to the bank, meat-eaters. Convinced yet? Winkie face. Is my experience simply anecdotal or typical? Let's take a look at facts.

So, seriously, can we settle the argument once and for all?

Is sex better with a vegan or not? People for the Ethical Treatment of Animals weighed in, of course. As we've mentioned, PETA is known for its effective and memorable public service ads and increasingly, paid commercials that are always in your face. One of its most controversial commercials got banned in the 2016 Super Bowl. But you can still watch on YouTube. Look for it under the title, "Last Longer." I know that Dr. Kahn also described it, but let's go there a little more because it is so fun.

The ad shows a split screen of two couples presumably having intercourse among the strategically placed sheets. Couple number 1, and the guy labeled the meat eater, obviously can't sustain an erection or climax. He dies a mortifying quick sexual death. The woman storms off in frustration. The second couple labeled "vegan" is still dancing in the sheets moaning away until the end of the 30 seconds when a banner plasters the screen saying, "Last Longer. Go Vegan."

PETA has been trying long and hard, literally, to get a commercial like this on the Super Bowl for years because of the game's largest TV audience reputation. The latest ads cost 5 million dollars, or $166,000 a second for a 30-second commercial. Raising the money wasn't the problem. Getting an industry bought off by the meat and dairy industries to relinquish its choke hold on the truth and run the ad was and still is the problem.

But no matter. These rejected ads get almost as many viewers eventually on YouTube and other social media platforms.

If you search "PETA sex" on YouTube, you'll come up with a 2014 ad Super Bowl reject showing scantily clad women losing strategically placed clothing and replacing them with strategically placed produce such as pumpkins and asparagus. "Vegetarians" last longer is the message, then later, "Go Veg." You could spend all evening watching the PETA or PETA inspired ads on YouTube. But be sure not to miss the one called "Penis Inspired New

2012 Provocative Advert" produced by PETA UK. This is a classic with old and young men alike, fully clothed but somehow having the largest carrots, cucumbers, eggplants and bananas nestled in front of a "hairy" collection of lettuces and escarole all placed in strategic sexual organ locations. Once in awhile, a flash of a couple of limes and oranges, standing in for testicles, poke out as these wildly energetic men dance at car washes, on tennis courts and public streets. I don't know how PETA found a 2-foot long, flexible carrot that hung down from one of the actor's groin, but it was memorable. I'm guessing you'll replay that one a few times. The actors' plant-based sexual organs bounce all over in each quick scene as the message "Increase Your Sexual Stamina" is followed by the finale, "Go Vegan."

Information flies at us at warp speed. Research is always growing and changing. But just keep searching "Vegans have better sex" and going forward, the number of scientific papers can only increase. It's all about blood flow. As the research builds showing how wonderfully a vegan diet prevents and reverses heart disease, so it will continue to build in the area of sexual dysfunction. Big time. This is a huge trend that won't reverse. So keep Googling, my friends.

CHAPTER 7

If Sex is 95% Between the Ears, Why Being Vegan Matters
Getting Down and Dirty to the Nitty Gritty

I developed a survey to really get at the differences men and women feel before and after they became vegan. Some people chose to answer the entire survey. Others chose to answer only parts or summarize. Some of the answers gathered from others have been used in other parts of the book. It is clear from so many respondents that being vegan makes a huge physical and emotional difference in relationships and in sex.

Here's a summary of some of the typical answers. Yes, results are typical. Ask your doctor if plants are right for you.:

How long have you been vegan?

A: Vegetarian with no eggs since 1987, vegan since 1993.

How long has your partner been vegan?

A: Two years.

How was sex, specifically intercourse, for you before being vegan, for your partner?

A: For me, well, I wasn't having a lot of sex before becoming vegan, so I'm not so qualified to comment. When I started having sex, I was already a vegetarian with no eggs, and had been for a few years. I can say that being vegan gives me more confidence regarding sex because I've been told that I smell nice. I don't normally wear deodorant unless I know I'm going to be in an extremely stressful situation or am wearing polyester (which I tend not to wear), and people, not knowing this, lots of times spontaneously say when they hug me, "You smell good!" My husband also really likes the way I smell, and, well, it's not a product. It's just that my diet has been pretty clean for a long time, so I don't smell the way I used to. When I was on the Standard American Diet (SAD), I most certainly needed deodorant! (Ellen's note: A friend who served 4 years in the Vietnam War said the South Vietnamese routinely commented that it was easy for the enemy to detect Americans because of their smell, attributed to the foul stench of animal consumption and digestion.)

Did you notice any changes in intercourse or sex in general after going vegan? If so, what?

A: I was so close to vegan when I lost my virginity that I didn't...

Did you experience any emotional changes with sex after going vegan? If so, what?

A: Again, I was so close. More with life, though, which spread into every area. When I definitely wasn't hurting/killing anyone to eat, I felt so much better.

Do you believe that going vegan has created beneficial physical and/or emotional changes in your sexual relationship(s)? If so, what?

A: Well, in all areas (I don't know about sexual, for lack of before-comparison), my endurance has gotten SO much better since being vegan. I (sadly) barely even move, much less exercise, but if I do end up going for a walk or bike ride (rare), I can do it for such a long time, and am not tired. When I was veggie but not vegan, I trekked in Thailand -- was about twenty-six years old. I was exercising A LOT then. There were younger men, athletic (which I'm so not) on the trek, and I was always in the rear. Five years later, I was doing a more strenuous trek in Peru, and hadn't exercised in a really long time, but I was vegan. There were athletic young men on that trek too, and to my great surprise, I'd be effortlessly in front of the pack.

Any advice for non-vegans and how sex might be enhanced if they went vegan?

A: Life, in all aspects, is enhanced by being vegan. There is a deep joy in being kind to animals and the planet. Also, being vegan really does make people smell better. And feel better. I can't imagine having sex after eating animal products -- probably feeling bloated, enervated, gassy...so not romantic. Feeling underlying guilt about doing heinous things to fellow beings. I have literally cried so many tears about eating so many animals growing up -- so much blood on my hands before my wires connected regarding this issue. I'm so glad my kids are lifelong vegans so they don't have to carry this subconscious/conscious load....

Do you know anyone else whose sex life changed after going vegan?

A: Sadly, I don't know tons of vegans -- and have not discussed sex with any vegan friends except for you.

Another response: I don't want to embarrass my spouse, but before I met him, I was dating a man 17 years younger. Since my current husband is 5 years older than me, I suddenly went up 22 years in age and maturity in terms of partner. But the older (vegetarian, later vegan) man had a lot more vigor than the younger one! And still does! My first husband, an omni, was beginning to lose his "vigor" in his early 40s, but he ate a lot of fish and cheese. My husband is now mid-50s with no signs of slowing down in that area. It is an unexpected blessing to being with a vegan male, and I try to make this point with others as a selling feature, hahaha, without being too graphic. All about the blood flow and veins is right!

My husband is very shy and would never discuss his activities with others, but I feel this is an important point to make. ED is a sign of a faltering vascular system, as you of course know! It is NOT just normal aging.

Summary of Answers

The bottom line is that sex for both sexes is inspired on a deeper level than just titillations and porn. While the visual images are key to stimulating basic animal arousal, what makes humans different from basic animal instincts is that we have the ability to process, think and feel in ways that are uniquely human. We have the ability to override our most selfish instincts to have a good time and still focus only on the other using a vegan lifestyle as our common bond. We also have the ability to be completely selfish and choose how we live our lives based on our various needs for survival. If the higher good, trying to eliminate suffering on all levels is where our priorities lie, then what we wake up and do in the morning becomes a fairly easy decision. Who we hang out with becomes easier. Who we have sex with becomes a no-brainer. The dedication to "the cause" does become the glue that holds our partnership together. As much free time as we can find is funneled into the cause because we realize on a daily basis, how little time we have to stop the freight train of ruin to the planet, our health and animals. There is always more power in numbers, and hanging out with someone who gets that is the biggest, juiciest aphrodisiac you can imagine. As money might be an aphrodisiac to the power-hungry, fighting for our survival using a vegan diet as our common bond is sexier and more enticing than all the gold at the Federal Reserve. Remembering all the different ways your love has shown love and compassion to humans and non-human animals is a wonderful cement. It can become strong enough to stand the test of time with lots of sentimental moments to build lasting memories. More than a flash in the pan, those memories become a lifetime of emotional and physical snapshots in a family tree of convictions that define a life lived with purpose and fulfillment. Hop in the sack knowing you have done everything you can to make a difference in the world.

CHAPTER 8

The Weirdest Thing That Ever Happened Or the World's Worst (Almost) Vegan Date

This is such a bizarre story that as I started telling it, people kept saying, you have to write it down or sell the movie rights. As a television reporter and observer of life, I have seen lots of strange stuff. But this took the vegan carrot cake. At the very least, it is a strange story. If you believe in synchronicity, energy that we can't define, or guardian angels, this is one for the record books.

I include it here for several reasons. 1) Just because your guy or gal is vegan doesn't mean that it is a match made in heaven. 2) As more of us become vegan, there is definitely safety in numbers, especially as the vegan community becomes more connected. 3) You can never be too careful or diligent enough.

It was Thursday. During the day, I had called my then boyfriend to clarify ending our year-long relationship. He was vegan. But the usual... commitment phobia. You know the type, vegan or not. He had given me mixed messages over the year, and there were definitely "buying signals" that the tide might change. Despite incredible highs, the relationship had been in a downward spiral for several weeks. I had seen this often in aging men as they no longer needed or wanted to be in a committed relationship. What was the point? They weren't going to raise children, and perhaps after living decades in a committed relationship(s), they were finally enjoying their freedom.

This breakup really was more about him and his personal stressors than anything that had to do with us. Fluctuating between the no commitment mode to something more, eventually imploded our interactions. On Tuesday of this same week, he initiated the breakup on Facetime. By Thursday, I had some, "wait, are we sure we're breaking up?" questions and called him. Another 30 minutes later, we were done. Really done. There was no doubt. I was a blithering mess.

My only saving grace to the day was I had a date with a guy arranged by a dating service. Now you might be asking, why would a well-known, otherwise self-confident author hire a dating service? I hate the bar scene. I had moaned to a non-vegan guy friend, "I can't meet any vegan men!" He goes, "What do you mean you can't meet any vegan men?! You're on the lecture circuit as a popular vegan author! How can you not meet any vegan men?!!"

I answered, "What am I supposed to say? Break my professionalism at the end of my talk with, 'OK now if anyone out there knows of a nice vegan man for me to date, please come up and see me?' I can't do that." He reluctantly agreed, "I guess not." Especially during my working in television, I found that men were not above confessing that they were going out with me as an "arm piece." The celebrityness of going out with a TV star, or so they thought, was way more important than getting to know me as a person.

Deep down, I knew that this latest relationship in my current author life was the same. Too many comments had surfaced that led me to believe my lover's interest was more about the eye candy appeal and hanging out with someone who had written a book. Or four. La-de-freakin-da. I just wanted to meet someone where my identity would be anonymous; someone who had no idea about me, what I did for a living, or even what I looked like. Someone who maybe could support me in a way I had not been supported, maybe ever.

The dating service, which was not cheap, spent a great deal of time doing personal interviews both in person and with written compatibility surveys. The lower your score, the more compatible you are. On paper, anyway. The owner of the franchise bragged to me during our interview that she was making 6 figures. I didn't doubt it. Subsequent news stories talked about how as these services up their "success" rate, more singles who have the means invest in the dating services to fill the void of meeting truly eligible partners. The services are generally good about asking participants what they want for the long term. Is it just a companion for lunch or dinner or a movie? Or are there long-term aspirations for a genuine relationship complete with commitment and potentially marriage? Sadly, I was told, nothing would be asked of me or my partners about dietary preferences or lifestyle value choices other than religion. Asking whether you wanted your partner to show up for dinner every night, they felt was more important than what was being served on the dinner plate. Even more dismal, I was warned, "Forget about finding anyone in our local database who is vegan. There aren't any." OK, I thought. I guess I'm going to have to give this my best shot at selling my date, if we were to continue dating, on the many features and benefits of veganism. But maybe not on the first date.

Up until this point, I had met some very interesting, incredibly bright and successful (by western values) guys--we're talking CEOs even, who really were-- who had no problem telling the world they or we were using a dating service. Other guys I met through the service didn't want that out there feeling somehow as they put it, they were "losers" because they couldn't meet women on their own. Frankly, I valued that guys would be willing to invest their money in a service that could find compatibility matches way beyond filling out a standardized form the way the popular online-only dating services do. Without naming names, I signed up for some of the more popular online dating services, some of them vegetarian even (as close as I could get to vegan), and still got pairing options with 20 year-old boys and older women. Neither were on my profile. At all.

The local dating service had called me in advance to let me know that the latest candidate, Joe (not his real name), the potential date, had a very low compatibility score of 14. In other words...it should be a perfect match. Only one little glitch they said that didn't fit into my profile. They wanted to know if I would make an exception. I had put in my profile to only date guys who were divorced. Yeah, yeah, yeah, I can hear you saying, "You should have known better. You shouldn't have gone there."

But before rushing to judgement, the service went on---He was not legally divorced but legally separated from his wife, we'll call her Linda...a few short weeks or at the most, months away from paperwork being accepted by the court. Just a formality, the service said. Was I still interested, they asked? They ran down his profile. Retired CEO of a wildly successful company. Very fit. Works out every day. Likes dancing, movies, boating and many of the things I liked. Opera? Yeah no. That last one must have been the one thing where we weren't in synch. But otherwise, what's not to like? You can't have everything. What if he is really cool and I passed? What could possibly go wrong? And if it did, it was just one date.

We went to a posh fish restaurant that had vegan options. We closed down the restaurant 5 hours later after talking about everything. In retrospect, as even he pointed out, "You know so much more about me than I do about you. I feel like I did all the talking." OK, guilty. I was a reporter. I was born asking questions. So his dominating the conversation didn't seem too out of line with my role and position. But I had no problem answering his questions if asked. There weren't too many of those, though.

At the end of the evening, I looked at him squarely in the eyes and said that I had "violated" my rules of dating married men because the dating service said the divorce was imminent, only a "formality." "You're not planning to go back to her or anything, are you?" I asked. "Oh no," he insisted without missing a beat. He did say that Linda became vegan while he was married and perhaps, I could get him to go vegan too. Yeah, vegans, especially vegan chefs and authors get that a lot. I'm so over being anyone's free private chef.

The next morning he called and apologized for asking on such short notice but there was a national dance competition at the Ritz. Did I want to come? Not wanting to seem too easy, I said, "Sure, though if you'd asked me for tomorrow night, I wouldn't have been available." He said, "You'll need a cocktail dress." Coming out of a previous marriage that involved sailing, running, and living and pretty much staying on our 7 mile-long island, I didn't own a cocktail dress. I wasn't even sure what the definition of that was anymore. I lived in running shorts, running shoes, running shirts and bathing suits. When I wasn't wearing running shoes, I wore flip-flops.

I knew that I didn't want to spend hundreds of dollars and went to a second-hand store where I found a cocktail dress for $7 and a pair of 2-inch heels for $5. I hadn't worn heels like that since I'd moved to Florida in 2003. I remember at a runners club annual dinner when all the women in the bathroom bemoaned having to wear heels to the event. Runners don't wear heels because they reposition our knee caps and as a result, they kill our knees. The heels I bought were purposely a size too big so that my bunions wouldn't be cramped. But when I went to get in the car, one of the shoes slid off Cinderella style. I giggled and tried to make a joke of it.

The dance competition was fabulous. In the ballroom with full dancefloor and stage lighting, the floor was surrounded by round tables where we sat at in the front row. It was right out of "Dancing with the Stars," except the colorful, glittery costumes were in your face, as were the superfit 20-something dancers. All of a sudden, my 103 5K age group awards seemed completely insignificant. My 6-pack abs and core felt like mush.

3 hours of this was interspersed with a few small breaks in which the audience could dance with an instructor or each other. Before we got in the car, I had asked Joe if we would be dancing. He said no. So I wore the secondhand store heels. They had no straps. I had to scrunch my toes to make sure the shoes stayed on when I walked. Of course, once we got to the competition, there were breaks throughout the evening when the dance floor was open to the public. I really had to scrunch my toes to keep those shoes on when we danced. I had totally forgotten how to wear heels. On the dance floor, I felt like a clod, praying that my shoes stayed on and my impinged ankle nerve wouldn't make my foot give out. I was struggling to stay balanced, let alone trying to remember 8th-grade fortnightly dance lessons in the foxtrot and cha-cha.

The whole night was a fairytale. Joe went to get his car out from the valet, who he tipped extra to have the car parked right in front. I half expected a pumpkin to arrive. I shook my head again, feeling like I was living some out-of-body fantasy. I thought at best, it was a great distraction from the events earlier in the day. Deep down, I knew I had just stepped into some white privileged daydream that would never suit me. I could hear my parents reminder, "Money doesn't buy happiness."

Because Joe lived 40 minutes away and the dance competition was near his home, I had offered to drive to the Ritz to meet him there. He insisted on coming to pick me up because as he put it, "Since it will be late at night when the competition ends, I would follow you back home to make sure you got home safely." Wow, I thought! Chivalry is not dead. Who does that in today's world?

We got back to my Gulf of Mexico condominium which was right on the beach. I invited him up, we drank some water, and then I asked if he wanted to take a walk on the beach. We walked for about an hour, talking about stars, and mostly about himself, before we went back to his car, where he got in and he drove home. He texted me several times on the way home and at home saying what great time he'd had.

Two days later, on Sunday, I got up and ran 10 miles in the rain with friends from my running club which always meets at the nearby beach. A tropical system kept a steady rain on us. I had committed to attending a late lunch at an Indian restaurant for our local veg meetup group about 30 minutes away.

During this entire time, I kept thinking of that last line in so many of my TV consumer reporting stories. I would close with the classic advice, "If it seems too good to be true, it probably is." I must have thought that a dozen times over the weekend, in wonderment, smiling. My smile would soon fade.

The short story is that at this meetup, a guy across from me at lunch mentions the dance contest at the Ritz. "Did you all hear about it?" he asked. Freak coincidence #1. Me: "I went to that."

Woman next to guy (Freak coincidence #2...that she is sitting across from me at a table of 30 vegans and vegetarians. If she or the guy had been sitting anywhere else, the following conversation would not have occurred): She goes, "With Joe?" Me: "Yes. How did you know?"

Woman: "He's my husband." (Freak coincidence #3) "I went to the contest the next night, last night (Saturday) with another date." Grabbing her phone, here's the text Joe sent me saying how hot I looked. We're having a date tonight. We're going to a movie. My mouth drops open as I see his text to the wife he is supposedly divorcing and never getting back together with again.

The table, along with me, is riveted, stunned and quickly silent as the story unfolds before all of us, in live time, many agreeing that it is a def a movie. Like a game of the old "telephone," word spreads down the long rectangular table what is happening. Most eyes are staring in our direction. Everyone seems incredulous, mostly me, that this drama is happening live, in front of a vegan-friendly audience.

As sad as I was, I was so grateful to have avoided weeks, months, maybe years of grief. I should have trusted my instincts as I heard Joe plan out loud what temperature the house would be set at, what dresses he would buy me, and how he might go vegan "this time" if I cooked some vegan meals in his new home that he was still building. Linda gave me the address. I drove by and saw the multi-million-dollar monstrosity overlooking Sarasota Bay. Ah...it could have been mine. Let it go, I chided my most non-greedy inner voice.

What were the odds that the Universe would place his wife next to me in a group of 30+ people, within hours of my being taken with (talking only, fortunately) with her hubby? I just have to ask...why, male species, why?

Those sitting closest to Linda and me at the Meetup were the most caught up in the drama. Two of them insisted on us telling them the next chapter as soon as we knew it. They goaded us to "play" Joe somehow. But neither of us wanted to do that. Although Linda did call me the next day (Monday) to tell me how her movie date with Joe went.

She told me that she wanted to keep being friends with him, but that I could "have him." She had shared with me that Joe fully expected I would give up my career to be with him, as Linda had. In fact, Linda said that part of her divorce settlement was an undisclosed amount of money for alimony. She had given up her lucrative career to be a stay-at-home chef and housekeeper in Joe's large house. She traveled with him. She told me that Joe expected I would let him keep eating his meat in a "Kitchen Divided" per my book by that name I had given him. She said she asked Joe, "But Ellen travels the country on weekends speaking at Vegfests." "No problem," she said he quipped. "I can travel with her or I can stay home and watch football." He had our life completely mapped out after only 2 dates. I have never been so astounded. Is there no man on the planet that could like/love me for what I do and who I am without wanting to change me into a tennis-playing, Pinochle or bridge-playing, Florida retiree? I digress. Though I must confess that I have started playing Pinochle with my newest friend and love the mental challenge.

On her date, Linda did not have the courage to tell Joe that she and I had met. But she fully expected that I would share our meeting as my reason for not continuing to go out with him again.

Linda and I last parted on the phone with cheerful giggles, and agreed to take dancing lessons at her favorite studio at the end of the week. I told her again that she could have Joe all to herself. She assured me she didn't want him and repeated her belief that he had joined the dating service to make her jealous.

As you might expect, I never heard from her again and have no idea how their story ended. I've had many synchronistic and weird things happen. Though I'm not one to believe in the supernatural, it is hard to believe that my parents, who always looked after me in so many cute and loving ways, didn't have something to do with this from heaven where they both currently reside.

Oh yes. I did text Joe after I spoke with Linda by phone that last time. Thank goodness for texts which keep a beautiful transcript of how life unfolds in the most bizarre moments. At least I had the presence of mind to take a selfie of Linda and me at the lunch. I sent Joe the selfie along with this:

Ellen: Who woulda thunk? I asked you last Thursday if there is any chance of you getting back together with your wife. Not at all you said. Just a formality of paperwork which would happen soon. The dating service told me the same. So I believed you.

Then you text your wife to tell her how hot she looks Saturday night. And you go to a movie with her Sunday night. Who hires a dating service and then goes out with their wife 2 days later? Trying to make her jealous?

How do I know this? Because some guy across from me at the vegan meetup on Sunday afternoon decides to talk about dancing at the Ritz. I piped up, "Oh I went to that Friday night." The woman next to him goes, "with Joe?" By the most bizarre set of circumstances that confounded everyone who was in earshot of that conversation, I went to one of the very few vegan meetups I ever go to in Sarasota, and happened to sit next to Linda. She's lovely. I hope you have a long life together. I was going to tell you in person, but the attached pix should tell you all you need to know. She didn't set it up (as she feared you would think). I just happened to walk into the right place at the right time with some guardian angel watching over me saving me from heartache. You seemed charming enough, though as you pointed out, you did almost all the talking.

I figure why waste my time. Believe it or not, some women don't give a hoot about money and do their passion because it's the right thing to do---with or without a man in their life who supports them emotionally. I'm a nice girl with solid midwestern values. I won't be bought by anyone. It was a fun fantasy for a couple days until I learned the truth. Honesty is what I have built a career on. My unusual energy and life's work are not for sale. We're done.

Joe: Whoa girl have you jumped to the wrong conclusion

    If you want to be done fine

    I told you I am friends with my X

    We danced for 10 years together including amateur competition

    I was happy to see her at the Ritz Saturday and she sat at another table

    Yes we went to a movie Sunday which we do once a month to catch up

    I'm not embarrassed by it I'm sorry you can't understand it.

    But my X and I are done as a couple

Ellen: I went through the same process a year ago. I know that if you agree on everything, the divorce can be final within a month. It would appear that you are nowhere near that and need time to put distance between that relationship and others. The dating service and you made it sound like it was very close to being done, which was why I violated my rule of not dating married men, no matter the circumstance. Not interested. Wish you the best.

Joe: Again your wrong all the papers were filed 2 months ago

    We were told it could take 12 to 14 weeks for final judgement

    I'm not trying to convince you

    I'm just stating what is fact

    I never would have started dating If I thought there was a chance of reconciliation

    Last thing I want to do is hurt another person

Ellen: Let me know when the divorce is final.

Joe: No problem

As of this writing, it's been a long time since that exchange. I am not holding my breath that the divorce will be final anytime soon. And even if I did become final, trust is an easy thing to lose and in some cases, impossible to regain. My bad. I should have held my ground with the dating service. Lesson learned. Just because someone is vegan, or vegan-friendly, doesn't make them a class act. It doesn't make them relationship or marriage material, as tempting as it might seem.

I grew up in a house where great values were taught, especially that money can't buy happiness or love. In my heart of hearts, I really do believe that. However, when I have stated this value throughout my life, some people respond with, yeah… but it sure can go a long way toward giving you happy moments, making you feel comfortable and providing a launching pad for the things you really want to accomplish in life.

I have spent periods of my life, dirt poor. Really dirt poor. I went to a college in California and hung out with a guy my parents didn't approve of. So I took on 3 jobs and continued to support myself and pay for tuition. It was a lesson in sticking to your principles. But many of us still want to win the lottery, wait for that vegan ship to come in, and, yes, be rescued by Prince Charming. I cringe as I write this from under my long-fought-for women's rights perspective, but yes, especially as we age, the fantasy or desire to be taken care of, both with women and men, can creep into our thinking on a subconscious and conscious level. Injury, trauma and loss, which increases in odds with age usually grabs us and makes us even more grateful for what we have. But it also makes us realize how short life can be, and how it can be taken away at any moment. The feeling of wanting to be taken care of is a normal and natural feeling, especially in times of stress and loss.

Personally, you may wonder, how does someone, who, seen by many as the epitome of independence, self-reliance abounding in endless physical and emotional strength say that? If I've heard it once, I've heard it a thousand times in my life..."You're SO strong." Yes. That's true. But we all have our crash and burn moments. We flame out. As activists especially, we can't see one more hateful post, one more abused and neglected animal, one more relationship crashing and burning from addictions of drugs, alcohol, and sex. Some days, my fellow activists, don't you just wake up and for once want to say, "Somebody, please take care of me today? Make it so I don't have to worry about animals, the planet, my parents, my kids, my family, my health, my pets, my money, the president or anyone else. If one more person calls me or someone else a name, or uses hateful and bullying speech, I'm signing off of Facebook." It would just be so much easier. And that actually may be a healthy thing to do. Activists will often say they're closing their account or taking an electronic holiday for a few days to refresh and regroup.

Despite the memes that challenge us to believe that nothing in life worth fighting for comes easy, some days we just want and need an "easy" button. Alas, we have arrived at the threshold of activist title and relationship burnout. Sticking our heads in the sand would be a relief. A welcome, warm vacation. But then we regroup and refocus and jump back on the activist trail, however each of us define that. The planet and the animals in particular, have no time to wait or for us to end our pity parties.

It is with that background in a demure daydream, I have fantasized, yes I have and please forgive me, about what a life with Joe might have been like.

I would have been so sold out. I suspect I might have convinced him to let me keep doing my vegan "thang" amid cruises and jaunts around the world. But those meal tickets come with a huge price.

Linda had shared with me that Joe had been having a long-time affair with another woman. That's just the way it was, she said. While some cultures and people can do fine with having multiple relationships at the same time, many of us can't handle that. Better to be alone and content with oneself than looking for another to complete us, right? The old adage of you must be happy with yourself first before you can truly be happy in a relationship with another, holds true almost without exception. In the end, every person decides for themselves. I don't regret the dating service experience. However, as of this writing, there are many more options for vegans, including local and national services that include eating preferences and are willing to match you up accordingly.

As it turned out, another guy I had been seeing for awhile and had ignored during the brief distraction with Joe, was much more real, honest and direct. His daughter is a chef and he raved about the plant-based meals she had prepared for him. During a 10-day visit with his daughter, my friend joyously ate her food, commenting that he could eat vegan even more. Was it a pure courtship desire to impress? Some of that was going on, I'm sure. But there was a real desire to explore the terrain, enjoy improved health and if in the process, it pleases me, so be it. I was game. Ultimately, as we all know, it is about pleasing ourselves first. Time will tell, of course. I am in no hurry to settle down, or just settle. Relationships can become so difficult as we age, whether you are in one or not.

As one friend put it, why would you even consider being in a relationship with a man after all that you have been through? The answer to that, as it must be with all humans who decide to partner up in some form or fashion, many other species partner up too. In species that don't give too much thought about that, it is mainly for survival, finding food for each other and taking turns guarding the nest. The term "empty nesters" evolved because even after child-rearing is done, parents still often stay together in other species as well as our own.

When the expression, "Until death do us part" was created, it was during a time long ago when the average lifespan was 40 years-old. It is a lot more difficult to stay monogamous for another 40 or so years.

In the months and years since my last divorce, I've read and researched in my usual fashion, exploring many sources on how the male and female brain and emotions work. Growing up in the sexual revolution, we were taught equality and that there really aren't that many significant differences between the sexes. Or that there shouldn't be. However, I had 3 daughters. My sister-in-law had 4 sons. They were all about the same age. When her kids came over, the boys would beat up and tear each other, furniture and toys apart. And sometimes, even my girls got drawn into the brawls as bystanders, one of whom, at the age of 5, ended up with stitches from a fall off of a chair. We joked that each visit ended up with $50-$200 damage. My girls, as best they could, tried to play quietly with their dolls, books and engaged in other more sedate activities. I resisted believing there was any difference among the sexes until I saw it play out. Into adulthood and multiple relationships, my observation is guys love to be physical, be it sports or anything in motion. When the going gets tough, generally, they hate talking about it. The fewer the minutes spent on talking about relationships or emotions, the better. If there's a problem, they prefer to run or engage in sports, go out to the garage or somewhere that allows them to build, or construct or otherwise fix a piece of furniture, equipment or a vehicle. Give them a few days or weeks to fix or landscape a house and bliss sets in. Help them with those projects in some small or big way, and they will like, love, or at least remember you forever. It is kind of all about anger and negative feeling management. I'm thinking that the guy who got so angry with me over my breaking up with him resulting in his punching a hole in my drywall could have done much better for himself and his arm by going out for a run or stripping some furniture. Who knows how much calmer he might have been if a vegan diet, known for taming the raging testosterone that men in Western cultures have too much of anyway, had been coursing through his blood.

My research also brings me to the conclusion that men are just programmed physically for multiple relationships. It's hard for them to really settle down and buy into the theory of one woman for the rest of their lives. Not to say it doesn't happen. There are couples like my folks who went 64 years. It wasn't until mid-elementary school that I realized that they both had different first names. It was a sad day for me when I was told that they both were not named "Honey" as I had put down on some school form. Having that kind of love and devotion as a role model can also be a tough expectation in the grownup world looking for relationships to be like that.

While some of what I have written has explored a few of the negative experiences of having high expectations of a vegan partner, and potential pitfalls involved are well worth the incredible highs of being with someone is so in synch with your values, goals and dreams. There is nothing like it, and you will know when you're there. You may have to kiss those few frogs to get your prince/princess. I would just suggest that you hang in there for awhile and know that if you want that vegan partner, it can happen. It may take walking through hell and back. But it is so worth it. SO worth it!

CHAPTER 9

The Male Perspective: Why You Might Want to Pay Attention if You're a Guy

This chapter is an attempt to include the male point of view in what it means to be a vegan in the emotional, physical and spiritual definitions. I have consulted my most trusted and favorite vegans. As promised, their identities are protected. They did not want to be associated as a vegan stud. Ah...men... not wanting to be sex objects. Who woulda thunk?

As for the emotional part of sex, men do see it as women often do-- 95% between the ears. Men often view being vegan as making them more sensitive, compassionate and receptive when it comes to meeting the needs of their women. They say being vegan makes them feel less goal oriented and focused on what pleases their partner. The word "compassionate," most often used by vegans to describe themselves, is usually associated with compassion for all animals. But with all the words and definitions "compassion" has listed in Webster's Dictionary, "pity, sympathy, empathy, care, concern, sensitivity, warmth, love, tenderness, mercy, tolerance, kindness, humanity, charity," what woman wouldn't want all that in her bed? Or in a man? Or a man wanting that in a woman? Or qualities friends of any sexual orientation seek in each other?

The ethic of the values of veganism--treating it more as a lifestyle than just a diet--gives couples a feeling of freedom and power at the same time. "Veganism transcends the physical," as one described it. "When both partners share the same values and ethics, it's a real turn-on. It keeps you in synch. Shared higher values makes you feel more erotic, and sensitive to your partner's eroticism. Altruism becomes the motivating force in your life. That can be very stimulating and never-ending. It doesn't get dull."

And another pearl of wisdom, "Serving the higher good is a real turn on and you're focused outside of yourself on other people and saving animals. The earth and your life become one of immersion in beauty. And that is a wonderful shared sensuality that never gets old. Higher shared values are more erotic. I want to implore people to go vegan and find a partner to share your vegan values with, and then every day becomes much more exotic and erotic. You get to re-create every single day because you're sharing a common value. It's exciting."

If we are more tuned into how animals think and feel, do we become more tuned in to our own animal-like behavior? Do we understand and connect our behavior better because we see how animal-like it is? Perhaps. If we are tuned into the non-verbals of animals, maybe we become more aware of how unspoken communication takes place between humans. When you care more about your partner's happiness, you sense their needs without them asking. You instinctively and almost intuitively know when they need a hug or a peek on their neck.

Stamina often refers to physical strength and endurance in sexual activity. Physical performance aside, many couples report that the common bond of being on the same wave lengths spiritually and philosophically puts them on cloud 9. They say that sex is 95% between the ears, or somewhere close. Because of that, for vegans, sex is rarely if ever, goal oriented.

However, couples report lasting longer for both men and women. It's about the immersion in the spiritual and the immersion in values. When these two emotional pieces combine with the physical, it is magical.

Here is one testimonial from a man who went out with a vegan for the first time. It was their first date, and it was the first time he had ever met, let alone, dated anyone who was vegan. He noticed her eating a large salad and a lot of vegetables. When he noticed, and then commented, "You're eating vegetarian, aren't you?" Men are so perceptive. She answered, "Why yes. Actually it's vegan. Nothing with a mama or a face." She had liked her date up until then and in somewhat typical female stereotypical apologetic fashion said, "But I don't shove it down anyone's throat." "That's good," he answered, not showing any inclination of wanting to know another thing about veganism. She figured, "OK, we're done." She didn't return his calls for a few weeks. When she did, all of a sudden, he was interested in knowing more about her and her lifestyle. What a difference a little indifference can make. She took him under wing and the vegan tutorial took off. 6 months later, here is the report from a smitten and changed carnivore:

"I spent the first seventy years of my life eating and enjoying meat, fish and dairy like just about everyone I knew. I was taught by my parents, teachers and church that Homo sapiens were meant to eat these things. I remember studying how our ancestors scavenged and hunted for their food. I learned how beef was raised and slaughtered for the benefit of mankind. Doctors and nurses including the national health officials sent films of the "Proper diet for healthy living" to the schools. The famous food groups were displayed in triangles for easy understanding. When I was about twelve my father took me to the famous Chicago stockyards to see the operation of thousands of steer being led to their slaughter. Several of my friends were taught by their fathers to shoot a gun and go hunting, fishing and trapping.

I grew up firmly believing that this was the natural order of things. Man was on top of the food chain and it was perfectly honorable to raise animals and fish for human consumption and mankind's survival. My mother even taught me how to select meat and the various cuts of meat that were available in the markets.

I did not question my elders nor did I even think about it until I met a special person who took the time to enlighten me. It was very difficult for me to grasp the impact I was making on our environment. I also learned what damage I had been doing to my body over the seventy years.

Now armed with this new insight I was faced with the task of unlearning all that I had been taught and undoing all my habits and tastes. Slowly, very slowly I entered into the vegan world. First I stopped eating beef, chicken, fish and poultry. Second, I stopped dairy milk and dairy butter replacing it with similar tasting vegan alternatives. Mayonnaise was the last to go. I won't kid you, it was tough to let go of what I thought was normal and tasted so good. I'm now a Vegenaise addict.

One of the things from my prior diet was peanut butter. I did not have to give that up and in fact, I ate even more of it. I learned about all kinds of plant foods that I shunned over the years and plants that I did not even know existed. I not only learned about all the alternative foods that are now available but I learned about the health benefits associated with a plant based diet.

As the months passed I found myself still desiring my old standbys. I would order a hamburger or put a steak on the grill or sit down to a perfectly prepared swordfish or salmon dinner. Much to my surprise that old familiar taste was different. It wasn't the taste I remembered. It was so much less than my expectations. The beef especially was almost revolting. Not only were my old favorite foods not pleasant but they gave me gastric and abdominal pain.

After a few missteps off the vegan diet I began to notice the benefits of a plant based diet. I am not sure how to describe the symptoms without stating them in graphic terms. My sinuses seemed to dry up. In the past I would wake up in the morning and have to blow my nose two or three times in succession. I would spend the first half hour coughing up mucus that had accumulated in my throat during the night. Having been a smoker for over fifty years I was suffering from COPD and the beginnings of asthma. Once firmly on the vegan regimen I realized better breathing capacity.

The best benefit that I was pleased to discover was my sexual ability improvement. I started to believe that at seventy perhaps my youthful sexual prowess was naturally fading. I was resigned to writing it off as "old age." I found it more and more difficult to not only get an erection but sustaining it. If I was lucky enough to have an erection and begin a sexual encounter, I would run out of breath and out of energy before the act concluded. It was very discouraging to say the least. After about two months eating a primarily vegan diet I noticed that I was becoming more easily aroused to an erect state and that I could sustain the erection during a full and satisfying bout of lovemaking. I wasn't running out of breath and I wasn't tiring due to the physical effort required.

I became more energetic. I wanted to do more activities. I began cycling on a daily basis. I kept increasing the distance of the bike rides much to my surprise. I started feeling charged with energy. My attitude and outlook on life itself improved. I was no longer getting old. I was becoming incredibly revitalized.

On another note my prospective on my environment changed too. I have always loved and cared for pets and enjoyed nature walks and birdwatching. I even volunteered at the local animal shelter. I just never associated that love with animals that were intended for human consumption. I never even gave it a thought of how the steer, lamb, pig, chicken, turkey, or fish got to my plate, until I took the time to research it. What I found made me sad. I could not believe how the dairy, meat, and fish industries treat the animals and fish in mass producing the products for market. It is so incongruent the way we can love our little puppy and allow such mistreatment of other animals.

In summary, this has been a wonderful awakening of my mind and my body. A body that I intend to enjoy for many years more than I would have enjoyed under my old, unhealthy way of life."

Or this conclusion by a converted now sexually active vegan who had given up on sex for decades:

"After a man fails two or three times in a row, he starts to believe that he'll never have an erection again. It becomes a self-fulfilling prophecy that is very difficult to stop. This feeling of inadequacy is what the drug companies feed on to sell their ED drugs. And if you go vegan and get off the drugs, you won't need to build two bathtubs side-by-side outside. Or anywhere. Hanging out in one tub, inside, will be just dandy and all you ever need for those magical moments."

In the words of this recovering ED male who has not taken Viagra in almost a year after eating a 95% vegan diet (he's still working on those addictive coffee creamers and cheese served at social functions.):

"ED lowers the person's spirit. They feel less capable. They become less active. They feel less desireable to potential partners. They retreat into believing they are just getting old. The downward spiral begins and the rest of their health follows downward also."

Take heart that so many of these patterns and vicious cycles can be reversed and stopped. Just as heart disease can be reversed on a vegan diet, so can ED and all the benefits that can produce: more energy, stamina and a serious attitude adjustment filled with positive thoughts and much more happiness, in bed and out.

CHAPTER 10

How a Vegan Diet Affects Women and Sex: A Personal Story

Can Suicide Be Prevented on a Vegan Diet?

Dr. Kahn has addressed how having all your parts in working order can make life good in and out of bed. As he also points out, there are many causes of ED and issues that come up for men and women that have nothing to do with what comes up in 6 inches or 60 years of living.

In the darkest moments, the older we get, it is common to have regrets and second guesses, as much as we know deep down we shouldn't do that. But in wondering how life might have been different in a vegan world, one of the threads woven into my life has been depression and suicide.

I'll never forget sharing with my Jewish OBGYN once what was happening on the home front. He looked at me starkly after my recounting of notes I'd found filled with rants from an ex about depression and contemplating suicide. He said right out, "You do know that there is a higher incidence of depression and suicide in Jewish men, right?" I did not. His words haunted me, even until recently. At least one large study out of Israel supported earlier information that my doctor used in our conversations. Other health care professionals have told me they don't believe this is true and are not convinced by this study.

One of the most romantic relationships I ever had in my twenties actually found me engaged to the same man twice after we broke up once. I'll call him Sam. He sent me flowers all the time and we jet-setted around the Caribbean often when he wasn't working long hours building his career. There was something just not quite right that I couldn't pinpoint, and I broke the first engagement off, accepting a TV job in another state. He begged me not to go, and I broke down and decided to stay put.

We ate healthfully preparing huge veggie-rich salads every night after work, though we both ate fish. This was my first experience with a man with erectile dysfunction. He was only 28. He blamed the problem on everyone and everything in life, mainly his own insecurities. Was it the dysfunctional relationship he had with his parents? Was it diet, I would wonder later?

There were other familial issues in play, but his flash point to anger got him in trouble four months later when we accidentally missed a cancelled flight in the Virgin Islands. It was the airline's fault, and he got so mad, security had to be called during the days when security was never called. The scary thing was he totally blacked out during the incident and didn't recall it. He wasn't willing to get help, and I wasn't willing to gamble my personal life away. I called up the scorned news director from the job I'd turned down, found the offer was still on the table and ran. I'm so good at running.

Sam begged me for the better part of the next year to come back. He called and wrote to my parents. No one ever made such a play for me as Sam did. But the idea of him going around me trying to reach me through my parents didn't go over well. My parents made no secret thinking that this up and coming successful businessman was perfect for their daughter. And yet, as always, they deferred to my judgement delivering their frequent line, "Do what makes you happy."

Sam never married until about ten years ago. And as many people do, not long ago, I had an overwhelming urge to Google him in that moment of, "wonder what ever happened to Sam." Truth be known, I had Googled him over the years and saw that he had a very successful career, great home, improving lives, and in the photos I saw, he had a very long line of gorgeous women on his sleeve. He never had children.

I contacted him only once when I was divorced. It was the world's shortest conversation. He said simply, "Not interested." He eventually did marry a beautiful, successful woman, and I thought all was well. Until the first newspaper article popped up and I saw that he had committed suicide. I was shocked. I couldn't imagine what had really happened. The self-doubts rolled in like a tsunami. Had he still been impotent all those years? Despite his success as we define it in our culture, was it all a cover for those deep-seated insecurities that probably didn't resolve, and maybe even grew in a perpetual, vicious cycle of personal failure. I could only imagine. I will never know.

I assumed by the photos I saw of his increased girth, that his diet didn't remain as healthy as it was when I knew him. Did the ED and resulting depression get him in the end? Was there anything I could have done, I've asked a thousand times since I saw the article? Would a vegan diet have cleared out his arteries, his capillaries in his heart and brain to make life better? A vegan diet has been associated with alleviating symptoms of depression. Many studies show that vegans suffer far less than meat eaters from depression, anxiety, stress and mood swings. If Sam had gone vegan, could his suicide been averted? In 2013, a large epigenetics study conducted in Israel and the United States funded by the National Institutes of Health did in fact establish the genetic connection between manic depression and schizophrenia (split personality disorders) and Ashkenazi Jews. The study of 2500 Jews found the rate of both of these diseases at 40%, compared to only 15% in the general population.

A friend chided me, "Of course there was nothing you could have done. You tried. He rejected you years ago. You were so young when you had your relationship. How could either of you have known what you wanted, or could it have even lasted? If you had married, think of the heartache you would be suffering now." She was right. Our relationship may not have survived. I don't tolerate out-of-control anger very well. But this is one chapter that will always remain open with so many unresolved questions. Coulda, shoulda, woulda... I know that a vegan diet isn't a cure all. Heck, it didn't even help my flat feet. But there is so much research now supporting increased serotonin, the "happy chemical," with vegan eating. The 2012 study in the *Nutrition Journal* said:

Consuming fruits and veggies can effectively increase serotonin levels which can lead to the desire to have more sex. Those who don't eat any meat tend to be happier and less stressed than those who eat meat. The team of researchers attributed this to the presence of fatty acids, specifically arachidonic acid (AA) — an animal source of omega-6 fatty acids — which can cause mood-disturbing changes in the brain at high levels.

We definitely need more studies. I know of one vegan man who committed suicide, but generally, the vegan men I have known are, at least on the surface, happy spirits. More men tend to commit suicide, and more people diagnosed with bipolar disorder commit suicide at a rate higher than the general population. One could argue, many people choose how we leave this earth. We can choose to go by diabetes, heart disease or other food or lifestyle related choices that cause preventable disease. But I will always wonder about Sam.

Vegan men I know more as close friends and/or lovers, seem to be in better moods, too, as long as they haven't seen an awful video about animal abuse or depressing health conditions recently. That is a huge accomplishment, especially given our complex and often horrific world full of so many major problems with the environment and the animals, including us, who live in it. On the flip side, vegans often feel like they are doing the very best and the most they can to try to prevent or alleviate suffering of all kinds. That doesn't put us in some rarified air. Nor should we go around feeling superior in some way.

The awareness of depression for both sexes is huge in helping a partner transition to veganism. There are so many reasons to be happy the change is occurring. Stressing the positive, if you are a woman living with such a man, is important to not necessarily stifle or redirect feelings, but to try and put problems in perspective. If we are to have successful sex lives, the psychological trauma from the visual of animal abuse that we may witness daily on social media has to be compartmentalized and shelved for the short-term time being, at least long enough to give ourselves permission to have a good time for a bit.

As Dr. Kahn has discussed, while women don't have the large penis that men do, anatomically speaking, the clitorus is as close as we can get. We still have the same blood and fluids that flow into our vaginal areas that make sex a walk in the park or a bad, painful marathon. Knowing the mood and anatomical requirements needed to de-stress, both for yourself and your partner, goes a long way to success, however you define it. While we hold up the orgasm, the climax, as the pinnacle and measure of success, that is not always the measure of intimacy and success. There are many ways to feel close to a partner, and good sex is but one delicious component of an 8-course meal, including lots of sumptuous desserts, that can last a lifetime.

Of course there are no guarantees. But working for the higher good, putting the cause of animals and human health above everything else, will make your juices flow. If you are fortunate to share your life with someone, or groups of people who get this, the world will be a better place. And you're allowed time off for good behavior. In bed.

CHAPTER 11

Getting Real Personal:
Why Vegans Do It Better

Besides the obvious reason of better blood flow to sexual organs, there are other reasons why vegans seem to have the edge in sexual energy, enjoyment and performance. If you Google "vegan sex," expect no less than 14 million hits, most of which are super positive reasons why vegans have it way better. Of course there are the naysayers. But they are in the super low minority and the occasional article such as one in the London Telegraph is shy on research refuting the overwhelming research supporting vegans have it made, and heavy on the "when you don't have facts, use mockery" technique. For example, in this description, you can kind of tell the bias and agenda of the publication before the first paragraph ends, "male meat-eaters are shunted off as sexless side orders, whilst plant-eaters serve up the main course of culinary carnal delight." Nice alliteration, but weak on facts.

I am leaving the current research updates to my esteemed co-author, Dr. Kahn, who, as a cardiologist not only must keep track of current research, but also sees the truth every day on the front lines, the advantages and disadvantages, in the unlikely event there are any, of following a vegan diet. I've scanned the lay person's summaries online of the very best reasons why vegans have it made in the shade in bed. In my surfing, I came up with, get this, "5 Reasons Why Vegans Have Better Sex," "7 Reasons Why Vegans Have Better Sex," and finally "9 Reasons Why Vegans Have Better Sex." Must be something about odd numbers that are more memorable. Did not find 4 or 8 reasons, though one 6 reasons article popped up.

There is nothing odd about vegan sex, or the ease at which vegans seem to have more effortless sex than those guys who can't get it up, or gals who dry up like a cactus. Having been to mainstream doctors all my life, that has been the predicted, dire warning that awaited me at the end of my sex life, somewhere between passing my prime at 29, and the earliest onset of pre-menopause.

The bottom line is that if all these features and benefits of a vegan diet are in place, we're going to be feeling pretty fit, feisty and ready for action. This is science. It's not like we pulled it out of our brains with no corroboration. Let's extract some of the most commonly mentioned benefits in the literature, which is ultimately, why things generally go better with vegans.:

1) Smooth skin. A vegan diet rich in life-giving fruits and vegetables, with all their lush antioxidants, has been praised in books and elsewhere for decades as giving skin a glow. The hormones of dairy and fat-laden animal products which store the pesticides and other toxins very efficiently, ooze their way to the skin, the largest organ we own. You may know the overload toxin outbreaks as acne, eczema, and itching in places where the sun don't shine. Consuming water has been long documented for helping to support that glow that radiates from within. A popular book title, "Raw Food: 100 Recipes to Get the Glow," or a popular website and book, "Oh She Glows" are just two

examples of how the reputation of a vegan diet continues to be the diet of choice when it comes to overall well-being and feeling good about the skin you're in. If your skin feels good, you feel good and confident about your body. If loving someone else begins at home, loving yourself and all that you are and can be comes first. Fruits and vegetables are high in water content. So if you are consuming lots of those, your body will naturally fight off chronic dehydration which is rampant in our culture, especially as we age. We often forget to count those 8 glasses of water, or as the day wanes, we stare down those 64-ounce ginormous plastic water bottles. Eating a vegan diet will also improve the brightness of your eyes. The increased intake of vitamin C and antioxidants from all that plant intake means that your skin will wrinkle less and become softer, smoother and silkier to the touch. Your eyes will be whiter and sparkle more than they have done in years. Look at some of the older vegan doctors who have been eating this way for decades. Unfortunately, most of the doctors are male. But Drs. Neal Barnard, John McDougall and Michael Klaper, to name a few, look way younger than their years. Vegans often hear this. I often get "carded" when people hear how old I am. They at least go into some very animated exclamation such as, "No way!!!" and demand to see my driver's license. As I am very fond of saying, a vegan diet combined with aerobic activity such as running, is magical. Seriously, many people entering their golden years vegan-style are not slowing down. They look years younger than their counterparts and do all kinds of activities and sports that others their age wouldn't dream of doing. Results are typical. Ask your doctor if plants are right for you.

2) If your body is very happy with your water content, it becomes one effervescent production plant of delightful bodily fluids. Translation: you're well lubricated. As my own experience described earlier reflects, being lubricated, even as you age, is just not a problem. Menopause is not a death sentence or an end to sexuality. In fact, not having to

worry about birth control is often a freeing feeling and allows you to be who you want to be without the responsibility of your reproductive actions. Vegan foods can actually increase lubrication. The high water volume of plants such as cucumbers, watermelon and cantaloupe not only moisturize the skin, but along with omega 3 fatty acids such as nuts and seeds, they can be your one-stop shop for alleviating vaginal dryness. Creating nature's lube jobs goes a long way to increase self-confidence and ease for both men and women of your chosen sexual acts. While alcohol and caffeine may increase your sex drive by removing barriers and inhibitions, they are also dehydrating. So keep that in mind if vaginal dryness is an issue.

3) Some foods cause a chemical reaction in the body that increases the libido in both males and females. Some warn that vegans have a shortage of zinc. But zinc suppliers are in the plant kingdom. Foods with large levels of zinc and vitamin B complexes are said to elevate testosterone levels and boost sexual desire. Many common plant foods that are rich in zinc and vitamin B are: almonds, asparagus, celery, pumpkin seeds, chickpeas, basil, figs, pine nuts, avocado, and bananas.

4) You'll feel happier. There is more than one study that says focusing on compassion lowers your heart rate and makes you feel better. For example, a University of Wisconsin study measured the brainwaves of hundreds of meditators and found that when meditating on compassion, one monk in particular had increased gamma waves which are linked to attention, learning and memory, something that had not been reported in the literature previously. The study also showed that the part of the brain associated with happiness was abnormally large which crowds out the tendency to have negative thoughts. It is widely thought that humans evolved to have negative thoughts to keep them scared and focused on literally running from the wild animals that chased us. Taking pleasure in knowing that you are not eating wild or any other animals three times a day will go a

long way in chasing that tendency we humans have to go to the dark side.

5) Contrary to conventional wisdom, ED is not caused by anxiety. It is pretty much the result of a combination of physical and sometimes, psychological problems. The biggest obstacle to a hard penis is blood flow. Studies have found that up 3/4s of heart disease patients have ED. That is one loud canary in the coal mine screaming his/her head off. Not only does the saturated fat in meat restrict blood flow all over the body, but it causes increases in blood pressure. All of that makes it difficult for enough blood to find its way into the vessels of all our organs, including the penis and even the vagina, labia and surrounding tissues for women. All necessary for the act and everything leading up to it. Even the clitoris needs to get blood flow to rise to the occasion.

6) Plants go better with semen. And all bodily fluids, for that matter. The reason is, it is made up, in part, of vitamin C and zinc, abundant in plant foods such as citrus fruits for vitamin C, and kidney beans, pumpkin and flax seeds, and spinach for zinc. If you eat more fruit, bodily fluids will taste sweeter. Even chlorophyll in green plants such as parsley and celery sweetens the load. Especially pineapples, bananas and papayas. Google "Do foods affect the Taste of Semen" and 2 million answers pop up. Some of them are more credible than others. Part of the problem is that taste is a somewhat subjective sense to study and evaluate. Pretty much all we are left with are websites and the surveys they've conducted. The repeat offenders that pop up are: red meat makes semen taste salty. Bitterness in seminal fluid is associated with caffeine, cigarettes, and preservatives in junk foods.

Some websites say that ejaculate should normally smell like chlorine or ammonia. Maybe for meat-eaters. But that's not the experience of reporting vegans. Again, the Eat Vegan on $4 a Day mantra: there's no money in broccoli. And there's no money to be made in ejaculate aroma studies. One site suggested "masking" the smell with air fresheners, candles, incense and room sprays. Don't you just want to scream, "change your diet?" The simple "cure" for foul-smelling excretions is to eat beautiful smelling, aroma giving, colorful plants. In fact, any kind of drug the pharmaceutical industry might design, should there be a financial incentive to mask smells, is a guaranteed stink bomb in ejaculate.

Vegans don't get off the hook completely, although this is way less guaranteed than the stink from meat and dairy consumption. Vegetables from the sulphur-rich cruciferous or brassica and allium families can make semen taste a little like rotten eggs. Brassica vegetables include broccoli, kale, and especially potentially more offending cabbage. Allium vegetables include onions and garlic. But don't let these antioxidant powerhouses scare you away from the vegan party and the many benefits these nutrient-rich vegetables can give you. Garlic in particular, is associated with increased blood flow. In the big picture, meat-eaters' semen and body odors are far worse, according to many websites and personal accounts. Even a study by the investigative team at "Vice" took this on and confirmed the same, though they did not specifically study vegans versus non.

Eggs are far more offensive in the offgas department. You would think that eggs might make the body smell of rotten eggs by the time they make it on down to the colon in our 1-3 day transit time. If you eat more fiber and produce, your transit time will be on the sooner end of that timetable. While the rotten egg smell can occur with egg ingestion and digestion, the literature also suggests rotting fish is the more recognized telling smell of decomposing eggs in the body Either way, definitely not a win-win.

Animal protein and fats breakdown or "putrefy" in the colon. This breakdown produces that rotten egg gas which is not only stinky, but in research, has been linked to increased chances of colon cancer. Think of a morgue or a funeral home. When a person dies, somewhere before the dead person is sent to a final resting place, wherever that is, embalmers rush to the funeral home to preserve what they can so that the physical body is preserved enough for relatives to say goodbye, especially if it is an open casket. In a morgue, the body is refrigerated, much like food, until the time of burial, kept in a body bag so that no one has to look at the possibly already decomposing flesh. The same thing happens to animal flesh if we eat it. Vegans never have to remember these kinds of visuals again.

The colon is the final processing plant before the body excretes the remains in the form of a bowel movement. If you are already vegan, you know that the difference between the smell of your bowel movements when you were not vegan and your bowel movements now, is like night and day. Nasty, versus pretty much no odor at all. The same applies to body odor, ejaculate and the female version of that, the release of vaginal fluids for lubrication before sex. It's like a spring day after going vegan. Who needs a douche?

Website after website which did get into direct comparisons between vegans and non-vegans semen and bodily fluids had similar language: "Odor from vegans in our survey definitely smelled sweeter than our meat-eating colleagues." The expression, "putrefaction," popularized by some of the early vegan doctors, refers to the toxins released into the bloodstream and intestines which then finds their way through the skin. Further detail about the 2006 Czechoslovakian "smell study" Dr. Kahn mentions, compared armpits of meat eaters to non and the veggie group won hands down. The women in the study reported that the meat-eating men really did smell putrid. This is further confirmation from my friend who served in the VietNam war being warned by the South Vietnamese that soldiers from the North could smell the enemy, the Americans, from their strong body odor as a result of eating stink bombs.

CHAPTER 12

Vegan Aphrodisiacs –Why Is This A Thing?

Hate to sound like a broken record, but Googling is definitely a measure of trending topics. If you Google "vegan aphrodisiacs" or some variation such as "vegan aphrodisiac recipes," "vegan aphrodisiac dinner," "vegan aphrodisiac foods," and almost any other word you could attach to "vegan aphrodisiac," once again, you'll get millions of hits.

The word, "aphrodisiac" comes from the Greek word "Aphrodite," the Greek goddess of love and beauty. This term is applied to foods and drinks that are believed to increase one's desire for sex or enhance one's sexual experience. Throughout history, various herbs, spices, fruits, and vegetables have been called aphrodisiacs simply because of their physical resemblance to female or male anatomy, like figs, cucumbers, and bananas. Others have achieved this distinction as the result of the mental or physical benefits that they provide, such as mood elevation, increased blood circulation and muscle control, heightened sexual arousal, or improved stamina and sexual performance.

When it comes to aphrodisiacs, much of the information out there is purely anecdotal, but don't let that keep you from adding more aphrodisiacs into your meal preparations. As they say, "don't knock it till you try it," and they may be just the thing you need to make you feel more sexual and to get more going on in the bedroom department.

In a vegan-starved world, many of us grew up believing that oysters and other mollusks were the main and perhaps the only source of sexually enhancing foods, otherwise known as an aphrodisiac. Nothing could be farther from the truth. Many healthy vegan foods are loaded up with aphrodisiac qualities. Since we know that meat clogs the arteries like a bad plumber, the converse is true. Vegans take in more vitamins such as A, C, E and potassium without supplementing.

Below is a list of some of our favorite vegan aphrodisiacs, in addition to the main ones Dr. Kahn has mentioned earlier. One or more of these plant-based ingredients are used in each of Beverly's recipes, which appear later in this book. The following is for educational purposes only. This information has not been evaluated by the Food and Drug Administration and is not intended to diagnose, treat, cure, or prevent any disease.

Almonds: This nut is one of the earliest-cultivated foods and has been regarded as a symbol of fertility throughout history. In fact, the tradition of having almonds at a wedding began during Roman times—guests would throw the nuts at newlyweds. It is also believed that the smell of almonds incites passion in women.

Apples: This juicy and sweet fruit is hard to resist, and most of us know about Adam and Eve's inability to resist the temptation of "the forbidden fruit" that led to the couple's being expelled from the Garden of Eden. For women, eating an apple a day may help with increasing vaginal lubrication and sexual function and satisfaction.

Artichokes: According to Swedish folklore, women who were feeling a bit neglected in the bedroom would serve artichokes to their lover to help stimulate sexual desire and stamina. The French are also fond of the artichoke, favoring mostly the inner artichoke heart, which they incorporate into many dishes, as they believed that it stimulates the genitals of both sexes.

Arugula: This peppery-tasting, leafy green is also called rocket in England, and it's a delicious addition to a salad. Arugula also helps with promoting good digestion. The Greeks and Romans often associated arugula with the fertility god Priapus, perhaps because of its high Vitamin A and C contents' ability to increase the intensity of one's orgasm.

Asparagus: Touted as an aphrodisiac as early as the 17th century. Further, prenuptial dinners in 19th century France often included three courses of asparagus. High in Vitamin E which increases blood and oxygen flow to the genitals. Asparagus boosts potassium and folic acid, the latter of which is said to boost histamine production—a necessary component in reaching orgasm for both sexes.

Avocado: The much-beloved avocado boasts the famous, hourglass feminine shape. That being said, the avocado fruit hangs in pairs on the tree much like male genitalia. High in omega-3 fatty acids and potassium, as well as Vitamin B6, which is known to increase male hormone production. They are so effective, in fact, that Spanish priests used to forbid their parishioners from eating them.

Bananas: Regarded as a symbol of fertility by Hindus. A banana has a sensual shape, which is appealing to many, and often leads to the desire to ravage the fruit with gusto. They are chock full of potassium and B vitamins which are both needed to produce sex hormones. Additionally, bananas contain the male libido-enhancing bromelain enzyme.

Basil: This member of the mint family helps promote circulation and is believed to stimulate sex drive. In Moldavian folklore, a man is destined to fall in love with a woman if he accepts a sprig of basil from her. Basil has a wonderful aroma and is commonly used to make pesto.

Beets: According to Greek mythology, Aphrodite ate beets to enhance her appeal to others. The Romans believed that they felt more amorous when they consumed either the flesh or juice of beets. This may have to do with beets containing a high amount of boron, a trace mineral that increases the body's sex hormones, as well as tryptophan, which can promote a feeling of well-being, and thus elevates moods and sexual arousal.

Berries (blackberries, blueberries, cranberries, raspberries, and strawberries): These flavorful morsels are bursting with juice, making them the perfect sweet and healthy treat for nibbling on with your lover! Or nibbling them off your lover, very, very slowly. Many of the phytochemicals and antioxidants found in berries help with reducing inflammation in your joints. Berries also contain anthocyanins (a phytochemical), which give them their rich blue, black, and red color, and also help to reduce your risk of getting a heart attack. Daily intake of blueberries is associated with helping to prevent Alzheimer's. Strawberries contain quercetin that protects against heart disease. Also, the Romans associated strawberries with Venus, the Roman goddess of love, because of their heart-shaped appearance and libido-enhancing properties.

Cardamom: The whole cardamom pods and the ground spice (made from the tiny seeds inside) have a sweet and delicate flavor with floral undertones, which is definitely enticing to the taste buds as well as your other senses. Some people even like to chew on cardamom seeds to freshen their breath. Additionally, cardamom has anti-inflammatory properties that help to increase blood flood. Cardamom is often used to flavor cookies, desserts, and the much-loved, Indian chai tea.

Carrots: For some, it may be the phallic shape of carrots, and for others, it may be the sweet taste and vibrant hue that they find so appealing. Either way, carrots are a must-have for any kitchen, as this widely used and versatile vegetable can be used to make anything from beverages to savory dishes or sweet desserts. Carrots are also an excellent source of beta-carotene and aid in hormone production. For guys, carrots are a mandatory ingredient for sperm production.

Celery: A whole head of celery does have a somewhat phallic form that some find quite appealing. Also, many people think that celery has a scent which is reminiscent of androstenone (a natural pheromone), and eating it can stimulate the release of sexual hormones.

Cherries: Both sweet and sour cherries are packed with many beneficial nutrients, like folate, iron, magnesium, potassium, and Vitamins A, C, and E, plus melatonin, a hormone made in the pineal gland of your brain, which helps to regulate your sleep and wake cycles. They also contain several antioxidants that help to keep your skin radiant and youthful, as well as quercetin, which has antihistamine properties that can come in handy during physical exertion.

Chia Seeds: The miniscule chia seeds were highly prized by the ancient Aztecs and Mayans, and were a staple of their daily diet. Some of the noteworthy benefits of consuming chia seeds include decreased inflammation and joint pain, increased energy and stamina, and enhanced athletic performance—all of which can be beneficial in the bedroom!

Chile Peppers: Whether hot or mild, chile peppers and ground spices made from them (like cayenne, chili powder, and paprika) are great for adding a spicy flavor to your food, and they can also help spice up your love life. They are high in capsaicin, which has the ability to increase your circulation, pulse rate, and body temperature (often making your sweat), and this mimics the way one often feels when aroused or having sex. Additionally, capsaicin is great for reducing pain and inflammation in your muscles and joints. Chile peppers are also capable of signaling your brain to release endorphins that make you feel good and improve your mood.

Chocolate (also cacao and cocoa powder): Lusciously rich chocolate is a staple Valentine's Day gift for a reason—this yummy food is full of compounds including anandaminde (a psychoactive feel-good chemical) and phenylethylamine (a chemical that releases dopamine in the pleasure centers of the brain and produces feelings of excitement and happiness). It also contains tryptophan (another happiness-enhancing chemical), which is essential for the brain to release serotonin. Also, consuming the naturally occurring caffeine found in cacao powder, cocoa powder, and chocolate will give you more energy.

Cilantro and Coriander: In leafy form it's known as cilantro, while the seeds of the plant are called coriander, and both of these are used prominently in Indian, Asian, Middle Eastern, and Mexican/Latin cuisines. They both also have anti-inflammatory, warming, and expectorant properties.

Cinnamon: One of the most-commonly used spices, cinnamon is often called a "warming spice" because it stimulates both your body temperature and appetite, and for many, their sexual appetite as well. Using cinnamon may help lower your blood pressure and improve mental alertness, and sprinkle some on a plate to help neutralize odors in the kitchen or bedroom. FYI, cinnamon, ginger, cloves, and nutmeg are combined to make pumpkin pie spice blend, and the scent of pumpkin pie has been documented to increase penile blood flow by 40%.

Cloves: For thousands of years, people have been chewing on cloves to help freshen their breath, which definitely doesn't hurt when you're trying to get things going. It's very aromatic and often paired with cinnamon or nutmeg in recipes.

Coconut (coconut milk, coconut water, fresh, and dried): The water found inside a coconut has the same level of electrolytes as your blood, and it has the ability to balance the pH levels in your body. Coconut-based products are not only fragrant and delicious, but they are also rich in Vitamin C, lauric acid (which boosts immunity), calcium, magnesium, and potassium, and consuming them can boost your metabolism and blood flow.

Coffee: For some, the smell of fresh coffee alone is enough to make them feel turned on and get their juices flowing. Plus, getting a dose of caffeine can boost your heart rate and blood flow, as well as increase your levels of dopamine (the neurotransmitter associated with the pleasure response in the brain). Coffee remains controversial with its reputation of short-term gains for long-term jitters.

Cucumbers: Perhaps it's their phallic shape, or maybe it's the cucumber's scent that's believed to increase blood flow to the vagina, which has led to their rumored use as a stand-in for an actual penis or vibrator. Cucumbers also naturally contain silica, which helps to keep your skin vibrant and healthy, reduces water retention, and supports your connective tissues that help you stay limber and ready for action.

Dates: According to Ayurvedic teachings, eating dates will purify the blood and increase semen production in men. Dates are extremely sweet, which is why they are often used as a sweetener in recipes by raw foodists and those who limit their processed sugar consumption. Their natural sugar content is not only pleasing to the tongue, but it can also give you an energy boost, which can come in handy during sex.

Fennel: Fennel has a subtle, licorice/anise-like flavor. When it comes to cooking, the entire thing can be used; the feathery fronds (which resemble dill) are used as a decorative garnish, the crisp stalks can stand in for celery, the bulb is often thinly sliced or cubed (eaten raw or cooked), and the whole seeds or ground powder is often used to flavor savory dishes (most notably sausages). Some of the reported benefits of fennel include reduced inflammation, improved circulation and vision, boosting the immune systems, and reducing the signs and symptoms of aging.

Figs: In the biblical story of the Garden of Eden, the fig leaf was tasked with protecting Adam and Eve's modesty. Figs were also Cleopatra's favorite fruit and the ancient Greeks associated them with love and fertility. They are also very effective at increasing libido and stamina in both males and females due to the high level of amino acids, antioxidants, and flavonoids.

Garlic: This member of the onion family contains allicin, an ingredient that increases blood flow. In both Hinduism and Jainism, garlic is considered to increase desire, in addition to warming the body. It is well known, however, that this little bulb creates some strong breath when eaten—you may want to steer clear of it on a first date.

Ginger: Known as one of the top natural anti-inflammatories to reduce muscle soreness, it also increases blood flow to all parts of your body. Fresh, dried, candied, and crystallized ginger can all add a zesty flavor to beverages, salads and slaws, soups, stir-fries, and other savory and sweet dishes.

Grapes (grapes and raisins): Throughout history, grapes have been a symbol of romance, love, and fertility. Both the Romans (Bacchus) and Greeks (Dionysus) honored gods that looked over the harvesting of grapes, winemaking, and fertility, and it's said that orgies were held to honor these gods and the rituals that surround them. In fact, newlyweds would be given clusters of grapes, as many thought that their seeds would help to bless them with many children. In most museums, you'll find cultural artifacts often depicting the cultivation of grapes, as well as their consumption, like images of people holding or nibbling on clusters of grapes, or drinking the juice and intoxicating wine that's made from them.

Mango: This exotic and succulent fruit is hard to resist, and it's believed to increase male libido and virility. In India, it's customary to hang mango leaves above the doorway of a honeymooning couple's new home as a fertility charm. Mangoes are an excellent source of Vitamin E, which many affectionately refer to as a "sex vitamin" because of its reputation for increasing the sexual arousal of both sexes.

Mint: The fragrance of mint has long been considered a sexual stimulant, as it's refreshing and relaxing to both men and women. Mint also has antiseptic and anti-inflammatory properties, as well as being helpful in alleviating insomnia and headaches.

Mushrooms: The fungus among us—mushrooms are often found hidden amongst the foliage in the forest, which not only makes them hard to acquire, but adds to their mystique as well. Some cultures believe that eating mushrooms will give you increased stamina and strength, or even immortality. The aroma of mushrooms is often described as earthy, pungent, or funky, and mushrooms contain high concentrations of the pheromone androstenone that makes you more attractive to the opposite sex. Additionally, some people think that mushroom caps somewhat resemble the rounded head of a penis.

Nutmeg: The hard, yet easily grated nutmeg was highly prized by the Hindus, as they were aware that usage helped to sweeten their breath, and the warming properties of this spice often stimulated their sexual appetite as well. Use freshly grated nutmeg for the best flavor and aroma, and it pairs nicely with cinnamon, ginger, cardamom, and/or cloves.

Okra: In Africa, okra was once affectionately referred to as "lady's fingers" and they believed that eating them would ignite one's passion for sex. In India, they also have a similar belief that consumption will rejuvenate and activate sexual desire. These two different cultures may have been on to something, as okra is rich in magnesium (a natural relaxant), folate, iron, zinc, and B vitamins, which are all nutrients that help to keep your sex organs happy and healthy.

Olives (olives and olive oil): Plump olives and their fragrant and fruity oil are good sources of monounsaturated and polyunsaturated fats, which aid in blood flow and hormone production. They're both used prominently in Greek, Italian, and Spanish cuisine, as they believe that consuming them makes their men more virile.

Papaya: The lusciously, sweet flavor and vibrant color of papaya is quite enticing, and many believe that the peppery-tasting seeds have contraceptive properties. Papaya is also packed with Vitamin A, which helps combat cell aging.

Pine Nuts: It takes a lot of time and effort to extract pine nuts from within their hard pine cone home. In the Middle Ages, people believed that eating pine nuts would give them a healthy sex drive. These rich and oily seeds are high in zinc, and taste great when used in pesto and other savory dishes.

Pineapple: At one time, pineapple was used as a treatment for impotence. Pineapple is a great source of Vitamin C, manganese, and thiamine, as well as bromelain, which can help reduce inflammation resulting from arthritis, strains and sprains, and surgery.

Pomegranate: Some people believe the "forbidden fruit" in the Bible wasn't an apple, but actually a pomegranate instead, and it's crimson seeds are considered to be a symbol of abundance and fertility. Eating pomegranate seeds or drinking pomegranate juice can help to lower cortisol levels, as well as increase testosterone production for both men and women, which can heighten one's sexual desire. Pomegranate also has high levels of nitric oxide, which opens up blood vessels, and increases blood flow, and can increase genital sensitivity and reduce erectile dysfunction.

Pumpkin Seeds: Like many other seeds, the green and tasty pumpkin seeds are high in energizing zinc. For men, this can be beneficial for keeping their prostate healthy, as well as increasing their testosterone and sperm production.

Soy (soy milk and other dairy alternatives, edamame, miso, soy sauce/ shoyu/tamari, tofu, and tempeh): For years, soy has received a bad rap from the dairy industry. However, soy is wonderfully versatile and a great source of plant-based protein, which helps to lower cholesterol levels and blood pressure while boosting circulation. It's also great for the sex lives of both guys and gals. For women, soy's natural nutrients have been linked to less PMS and it contains phytoestrogens (plant estrogens) that can help with increasing vaginal lubrication (meow!). The benefits for guys are even better—soy has been found to lower men's chances of developing cancer of the prostate (a vital gland for keeping everything pumping in the bedroom). Researchers at Kansas State University found that soy protein was just as good as beef for guys trying to gain muscle mass, without the heart-attack inducing cholesterol.

Tomatoes: Interestingly, tomatoes were once referred to as "love apples," as many people find that eating the tender flesh and its released juices to be a very erotic and sensual experience. Many claim that eating tomatoes before sex may even help to calm your nerves and improve muscle control, and their natural acidity stimulates blood flow to the lips and mouth.

Vanilla: The floral and intoxicating undertones of vanilla are hard to resist, and one whiff of vanilla is often all that's needed to get someone in a romantic mood. It also can mildly stimulate nerve endings, which in turn can make sexual stimulation and sensations even better!

Walnuts: The omega-3 fatty acids found in walnuts can help ward off cardiovascular disease, erratic heart beats, and improve blood circulation. They're also high in protein, iron, zinc, as well as the amino acid arginine, that's absorbed and converted by the body into nitric oxide, which helps to enlarge blood vessels and enhance blood flow to the penis. Currently, researchers are using walnuts to treat erectile dysfunction, and they've even developed a walnut-based pill for use as an alternative to Viagra.

Wine/Alcohol: Wine is rich in polyphenols and antioxidants (like resveratrol) that can improve circulation and boost blood flow to the sex organs, which helps with increasing sexual arousal. For some, having a glass of wine or other alcoholic beverage helps to lower their inhibitions and enhance a romantic evening—but keep moderation in mind, as too much could lead to drowsiness or a premature ending to your night's sexual escapades.

CHAPTER 13

Exercises to Spice It Up

Oh wait. Did you think that the 200 calories you burn during an orgasm is enough for your daily, or weekly workout? For some, it might be all you need, want or can do. But if you want to keep your machine well-oiled and optimally functioning, you may want to think about the regular tune-ups needed to keep your motors and connecting parts lasting and running at age-appropriate peak performance over a lifetime. Of course, what is age appropriate is pure conjecture as we see the golden years in sight. I ponder that I'm often the oldest or among the 5 or 10 oldest in the races I do. I wonder, why aren't more women my age running or racing? The answer, I believe, is yes, that old and tired refrain, diet and exercise.

Keep in mind, I'm a crazed woman by today's standards. I watched my aunt die of breast cancer when I was 5, then 3 more immediate family members get it. I knew exactly what was in store if I didn't try to defy my genes and fight to stay in shape. While veganism is not a guarantee against all diseases and things bad, it sure helps on so many levels of physical and emotional health. When people ask me what they think is a cutesy question, "What are you running from?" I answer, "Disease." It is that simple. But running or being at the top of your game, whatever that is, takes warm-ups, cool-downs and maintenance. Athletes don't just run out on the field and start playing. While nature wanted to preserve our species making it pretty easy relatively speaking to create a baby, the more in shape you are, the easier and more fun it will be.

This book is not to say that a vegan diet keeps your juices flowing to the day you die. No matter what you eat, the aging process will thin membranes of the vagina and urethra. Cervical mucous can diminish. But there is much you can do to fight the aging process, so don't give up just yet. One study shows that years of yoga can be very helpful for women entering menopause, in fact, they hardly notice it all. Some yoga poses such as twists target the adrenal and kidneys, producing just enough estrogen to give you an extra edge. The benefits of any exercise will pay off the rest of your life, even if you quit today. Hopefully you won't, because use it or lose it is still a good rule to follow, too. All of this assumes you won't retreat into couch potato-ism immediately.

Exercises Specific for Sex?

Like Adam and Eve or our ancient relatives needed a guide for sex exercises? No they did not. Somewhere along the way, somebody thought that was a good idea as we've seen in the extreme tantric yoga exercises. But in case you're not up for getting your panties in a wad, or your body in a pretzel with your significant other, we're going to take it down a notch.

I wouldn't have thought there was a thing to add to this chapter other than generic advice: stay in shape, eat a healthy, balanced vegan diet and you're good to go. But then, the bottom fell out. Literally. As I've described, a prolapsed uterus can be the result of gravity and age taking its toll.

When I wrote Vegan Fitness for Mortals, I wanted to provide a blueprint for finding your passion and entry level position into whatever sport or activity appeals. Many newfound vegans who lose weight and recover health and new-found energy ask me, as a personal trainer, how do you start a fitness program after a life of sedentary habits founded in obesity or an inactive lifestyle? It is the same for sex. I didn't really consider that until after Vegan Fitness came out. I started getting calls from magazines who wanted stories on the best exercises for sex. I hadn't really given it serious thought, but when I did, I realized that many exercises that are good for keeping your innards in, are good for the bedroom. Or as one lover said, "I think that running is really paying off in the way you have orgasms and the foreplay before it." Makes sense to me. But when you think about it, exercises that maximize the gluteus maximus, maximize all muscles involved in quivering, shaking and reaching the mountaintop. We know that there are more than 600 muscles in the body, and when you have sex, you use every single one of them. I don't think there is much room for disagreement on that.

That said, because I have put so many physical and massage therapists' children through college just to make sure all the parts are working and continue to keep working, I have developed a routine of exercises based on my experience and training.

First and foremost, stay in overall good shape the best you can. In my ideal world, we would all adore running without having to listen to music, our anatomy would be perfect to continue to do so until you reach 100, and our weight would stay no more than 5 pounds above what we weighed in high school. Right.

Getting real, keeping your aerobic activity at an optimal level for you, whatever that is to at least maintain a healthy weight, is critical. Many runners do so because you burn twice as many calories running as you do walking in the same amount of time. Add some green tea, coffee or other source of caffeine and your resting metabolism will be optimal, and if you need to lose weight, you might find the extra stimulants will help fuel that fire too. But stimulants also can stimulate the appetite. Of course, tea companies have all kinds of blends that suppress the appetite, but as much as possible, stick to natural methods of weight loss without adding artificial methods. It is still calories in, calories out. If you exercise and burn calories, you get to subtract those from your daily totals that maintain weight. But you also want to maintain good muscle mass, either through weight or resistance training, or dynamic muscle training. The first two, weight and resistance training are more static in nature. Think bench and leg presses, free weight arm curls, and resistance bands you can use attached to various body parts and appendages. Dynamic training is using force, sometimes explosive force to build muscles. Think walking lunges, skipping with arm circles and pogo hops. All of that will build muscle. The faster you work out, the harder your heart will work, and some people are able to accomplish both an aerobic and weight-training workout at the same time. But it's probably better for most of us to keep the two separate; better in terms of maintaining a healthy weight and not overdoing our workouts which can lead to repetitive motion injuries and burnout. It's important to not lose interest before you accomplish your goals.

Exercise conventional wisdom has evolved from spot training to sculpt your body to developing an overall plan. Gone are the days where doing isometric exercises will give you a flat belly. They won't. However, as I've outlined in the many workout programs in Vegan Fitness for Mortals, core strength is key for not only maintaining being able to run and place in hundreds of 5K or longer races like I have, but it is also critical in maintaining all the muscles that have anything to do with achieving an orgasm or foreplay leading up to it. I have videos on my YouTube channel of the most important exercises I do before I run, and cool down exercises and stretches after I run. These are the workouts that have kept me injury free through almost 40+ years of running and being a gym rat. I don't do all of them every time I run, but most of the time. They are a compilation of workouts from coaches over the years as well as watching my daughter's track team workouts. At 5 feet tall, she broke her high school pole vaulting record. She accomplished that through sprinting (OK, maybe a little genetics going on there) and through her love and gift of gymnastics. That got her on the University of Southern California's track team, where I had the pleasure of occasionally watching her workouts. They were kind of like my workouts, on steroids. But the same motions, just not the more tame and limited range of motion I did and still do.

Combined with physical therapists who thought my uterus was about to drop on the floor, along with the best of the best running exercises that will keep you toned in your private parts whether you run or not, I present:

Award Winning Exercises To Keep You Happy In Bed and Out

Ideally, you will have "warmed up" for at least 20 minutes, or a 1 mile jog or easy bike ride before doing these. Don't feel like you have to try all of these at once. Try a few and see how it goes. You may reach the point where you they are second nature and it isn't hard to remember them at all. You'll look forward to doing them to feel optimally warmed up before your workout and stretched after your workout. The goal is to get your blood flowing and moving into the larger muscles, including your heart, so that all your muscles will be happy to try these:

Warm-Ups

- **Circle Rotations:** Ankles, knees, hips, shoulders
- **Foot strengtheners:** Walk on heels to the count of 20, then toes, then walk toes pointed in, then out
- **Skipping:** high skipping to the count of 20, backwards, then forwards with 20 big arm circles forward, 20 reverse arm circles, repeat with small arm circles forwards and then reverse, 20 each. Take a breath. Skip forwards clapping hands up high overhead, then low underneath each leg as it is raised skipping. Repeat 20 times.

- **Side slides:** 20 in each direction.

- **Carioca:** Twist hips with top leg bending over bottom, then twist hips back so bottom leg becomes top bending over bottom leg. Do 20 in each direction.

- If you're in good shape, repeat carioca bringing knee closer to chest in an exaggerated motion.

- **Run with High Knees:** 20.

- **Butt kicks:** 20

Dynamic Strength Training:

- **Lunge and Rotate:** Arms twist to the outside in the "T" formation, 90 degree bend at the elbows. You should just be able to see them in your peripheral vision. Do 20 on each side, twisting to each side for each full count.

- **Lunge and Rotate:** Arms twist to the inside same as above.

- **Monster Walk:** Arms in "T," try to walk, touching one knee to the elbow on the same side. Don't overstretch

- **Pick Blueberries:** Take 3 steps. On third step, flex forward foot, lean over at waist with both arms and palms forward, as if scooping berries or shells off the ground. Return upright. Keep walking and on next third step, repeat above to 20 counts on both sides.

- **Over and Under Fence:** Imagine a barbed wire fence. Step over, then under. 20 times. Reverse in other direction.

- **Hamstring or Tin Soldier Walk:** Raise straight leg to opposite hand. Repeat to opposite leg and hand. 20 times.

- **Jumping Jacks:** Slow enough to land flat-footed (shin strengthener, shin splint prevention)

- **Seal Jacks:** Like jumping jacks, but arms more forward in front of chest, palms inward, land flat-footed. 20 times.
- **Gate Swings:** Jump feet shoulder width apart, toes, knees pointed out, press knees open with hands. 20 times.
- **Pogo Hop:** knees straight, arms at sides, 10 seconds fast
- **High Pogo Hop:** same, but higher, 10 seconds

For fun and extra challenges:
- **Skip Backwards:** (on a beach or somewhere that if you should fall, it won't hurt too much).
- **Lunge backwards**
- **Leg Swings:** If running, biking or other desired exercise, do up to 20 straight leg swings with flexed feet, holding onto a pole. Start facing pole, do 20 reps, switch to other leg. Then turn sideways to the pole, holding on, do 20 straight-leg swings in front, swinging to the end of your range of motion in the back.

Core Workout:

Windshield wipers: On back, bend knees alternate side to side with control 10 times each side

Scissors: Vertical shuffle. On flat back, keep legs straight and shuffle starting high at 90 degree angle to ground, drop low, returning high. Repeat 10 times.

Scissors: Horizontal. Small criss-cross sideways movements starting at 90 degree angle to ground, drop down, then raise up. Repeat 10 times.

Heel-Toe: Same position. Bent knees. Shins parallel to floor, do one leg at a time, touch toe to floor, then heel, return, alternate to other leg. Repeat 3 times.

Boat Hold: Curl up like a ball, low back, knees bent, shins parallel to floor, arms straight along legs, palms face up, then curl toward ankles, hold for 3 seconds, then back down to starting position. Repeat 5-10 times or until you can't.

Tabletop Crunch: Flat on back, raise both legs, keeping them straight at a 90 degree angle with feet flat and parallel to the ground, arms at sides on ground, palms down. Focus on raising lower back and legs into the air so that your abs do most of this movement, not the momentum of your legs. Lower slowly. Repeat slowly 10 times.

Baby Crunches: Curls and crunches get a bad rap, but if done correctly, they can help your supporting muscles just where you need them in a crunch, if you know what I mean. Knees bent, flat back, arms with elbows bent, palms skyward and fingertips just cupping your head, not for support, but for proper alignment. Eyes skyward, not at your knees, raise torso from waist only an inch or two off the head. Focus on this movement and not moving anything else. Elbows and arms stay put. Doing these slowly is better than speed.

Plank: Good for everything. Proper form makes all the difference. You can do this with straight arms, but if you have cranky, computer hands, your wrists may not be up for the party. So doing a plank with bent elbows works too. In either case, make sure your arms or elbows are directly below your shoulders. Toes are curled to support body which should be as straight as a plank. Start with 30 seconds. My personal record is 6:13 (on YouTube!) which is usually good enough to beat anyone I challenge at the end of my vegfest talks (with the exception of one very young yogini). But I hear the record is hours longer. I've yet to see it, though.

Cat Cow: On all fours, tabletop position start, inhale, allowing air to fill your lungs as you sag down like a cow. On the exhale, push body curling upward as an arching cat. Repeat doing movement to your breathing 10 times.

Fire Hydrant: An old standby, but works. From all fours, lift one bent leg as if you were a dog at a hydrant, extend the leg straight, bring it back to the bent-leg position and then down to all fours. Repeat on the opposite side. Complete the set 10 times.

Table Top Kicks: From all fours, extend one leg straight behind you, turn your head and as you look at your foot, swing your foot toward your waist in a side kick. Bring it back down to almost the starting position, but keep the leg straight and don't touch the ground. Repeat on that side 10 times. Switch to the other side for a set of 10 repetitions.

Nitty Gritty Sex-Directed Muscle Exercises

Perhaps since you read the part about my mainstream doctor sending me to a "sex physical therapist," you've been wondering what those exercises were about. Keep in mind, for a woman, this is all about keeping your pelvic floor tight enough to support the load. Women who have had natural childbirth may be more at risk, although having joyously done that, I wouldn't recommend that a fear of loosey goosey pelvic muscles later in in life prevent you from that experience, should you desire it. As an accredited La Leche League leader (breastfeeding information and support nonprofit), natural childbirth is way more beneficial for mom and baby, if you can do it. Most women can. We just need support and correct information to do so. The fact that there even exists such a speciality, pelvic floor physical therapists, tells you that this is quite a thing, even in the small town where I live.

These are good for both men and women, by the way, especially if you value your prostate, urethra, sphincters and other muscles that control "flow" of your lower body bodily fluids.

Kegels: Ewwww. Just when you thought you had had your last child, and you were done with these seemingly endless and boring rehab repetitions that are oh-so-good for your urine flow, they're back. No sweetheart, that was just the beginning. They never left. Or should have ever left.

Work up to doing 100 fast. Then 20 long-hold kegels, starting at 10 seconds, working up to 20, then 30-second holds for one. Release for just as long as you hold it, then start with the next one. They even sell kegel balls and devices, beyond dildos, now that you can squeeze in your vagina. But that seems like overkill, overpriced and who needs all those chemicals used in these devices and toys that are now being called into question? Go au naturale! Use your imagination. Or better still, get a real guy! Or gal.

Bridges: Flat on back, knees bend, push your glutes up, through your heels, until there's a straight line all the way from your bent knees to your chest, or even shoulders if you can comfortably lift that high. Hold for 20-30 seconds, then slowly lower. Barely touch the ground, then pop back up and hold again. Do 10-30. Feel those glutes squeeze. Enjoy. Fantasize.

1-Legged Bridges: Raise into position as above, then lift and straighten one leg. Keep breathing, hold for 10, lower leg, then switch to the opposite leg. Do both legs as a set, 10 times.

Belly Press Clock: Flat on back, bent knees. Put index finger of one hand right below belly-button. Imagine this is 12 on a clock. Raise belly, pressing into finger. Hold for 10 seconds. Move finger to 3 o'clock. Raise bell into finger, hold for 10 seconds. Do the same at 6 and 9 o'clock. Repeat each rotation 20-30 times.

Sheet/Towel Crunch: This seems kinky, but it's great for your core and innards. Do a baby crunch exactly as described above in "Baby Crunches." The difference will be, wrap a long beach towel or bed sheet behind your back, and twist it comfortably around your waist at the belly-button. As you crunch up, feel your muscles around your waist, push into and resist the towel. Repeat 10-30 times.

Flexibility Pays in Bed

Saving the best for last. While I never did gymnastics, all three of my children did with no stage mom pushing them. They loved, thrived in it, and coaches said they all had Olympic potential if their petite bodies and powerful minds wanted to take them there. I allowed them to compete to a certain level, but encouraged them to be well-rounded knowing that injury in gymnastics was common and longevity short. 2 of my daughters have just trained for a half-marathon together and all enjoy fitness activities. Point being, along with the running, they seemed to have inherited some flexibility genes. A physical therapist treating me once said, "the problem with you 'bendy' people is that your real risk is overdoing. You think you can pretty much do any yoga position and if not properly trained or warmed up, that's when you get injured. And indeed, I would say that of the very few injuries or discomforts I've had, yoga overdoing it was my most common culprit. The other risk is that our ligaments get overstretched like a rubberband. All of a sudden you're on top of a guy bouncing around like a bosu ball and you hear and feel that hip pop. At first, it doesn't hurt and nobody's concerned. Then when it does, like any overuse injury, you have to back off and regroup.

Remember to start slowly and just pick a few of these that seem manageable and build up. Worst thing is to get a case of the terrible toos-- too much too soon.

So...the best prevention against injury and stiffness (of the wrong kind) in bed is to be healthfully flexible. These are cool-downs and stretches I use in running, but many of them are yoga adaptations and good for whatever stiffness ails you.

Stretches

From a standing position:

Calf Stretches: Standing a foot or more from the wall, toes pointed toward the wall, feet 6 inches apart, lean toward the wall and support yourself against the wall with hands only. Keep heels on the ground, and bend one knee allowing that heel to come off the ground. Push with your hands through your heel to feel the stretch in the heel. Some people need to turn their back foot toes inward to really feel the stretch. Hold for 20-30 seconds. Don't feel the burn. Switch legs.

Hamstring Stretches: Find a wall, post, branch or something that is about a foot or more off the ground. Facing it, lift one leg, foot flexed, and gently lean forward from the waist as if in a swan dive. Reach the end of your comfortable range of motion, hold for 20-30 seconds. Repeat 2 more times. Switch legs and repeat.

Quad Stretch: Grab onto a post or wall with one hand. With the opposite hand, grab the heel counter of your shoe by bending at the knee. The key to feeling this one is squeezing your glutes tight and standing up straight gently to increase the pull you'll feel in your quads. This should feel good. Well, in theory, all of this should. Hold for 20-30 seconds. Switch to the other leg and repeat. You can repeat this exercise 1-2 more times per leg. Don't overdo, torque the knee or stretch the knee too hard.

Lower Back Stretch: Standing up straight, brings arms out to the sides, palms up, inhale to palms touching overhead. Twist hands so palms at 180 degrees facing outwards and allow arms to remain straight and fall away perpendicular to your body in a forward fold. At the same time, bend forward in that swan dive position allowing your arms and body to rest in a ragdoll position. Hang there motionless, grab your elbows, or let you arms sway from side to side from 30-60 seconds. Whatever feels good. Stand up slowly and repeat if you like.

Groin Stretch: Feet shoulder width apart or as wide as your comfort level permits, slow put most of your weight on one foot, lower upper body from torso and come to rest on your inner thigh with your hand or elbow, whatever reaches. Allow body weight to rest mostly on the one side leaning into the elbow. Hold for 20-30 seconds so that you feel the upper inner thigh stretch. Switch sides.

Downward Dog: From a standing position, swan dive to a forward fold, then reach hands toward the soft ground or mat in front of you. Your body should form an even and straight upside-down "V." Try to reach both heels to the ground, then alternating one heel at a time, pressing through as much as you can without overstretching the heel. "Walk the Dog" alternating pressing down each heel back and forth for about 30 seconds, taking a break and doing more walking if your heels can take it.

Pidgeon: From Downward Dog, lift one leg straight behind you keeping it as close to the same plane as your upper torso. Then slowly bring your leg under you and bend at the knee as close to a right angle to your chest as possible. You can stay right there, but if flexibility allows, sink down to the ground, staying even on your hips and lower your upper body, chest leaning forward trying to touch your bent leg at the knee. Stay there for 20-30 seconds. Slowly come back to Downward Dog, and switch legs.

On the Ground

Butterfly: Sitting up straight, allow knees to flop down to each side with soles of feet facing each other as much as your range of motion will allow. Grab your ankles with your hands and pull yourself forward to sit up straighter even more. Inhale slowly to the count of 20, then exhale, relax and repeat for a total of 10 times.

Figure 4 or Thread the Needle: On back, bend knees, then straighten one and grab behind the thigh above the knee with interlocked hands. Hold for 20 seconds feeling the stretch in the hamstrings. Then bend that leg, crossing the ankle above or below the other leg's knee cap, wherever you can reach. If you can, rest your elbow against the bent leg's inner thigh and press against the thigh, fighting the elbow's resistance. Hold for 20-30 seconds. Switch legs and repeat on the other side.

Remember that all these exercises are on my You Tube Channel. https://www.youtube.com/watch?v=KqgWJmRwlHU

CHAPTER 14

Resources for Vegan Singles and Couples

Not all that long ago, my Messenger box lit up from vegan entrepreneur Karine Brighten. A mover and shaker on the US West Coast, I was delighted to hear that she was starting a dating service for vegans, Veg Speed Date. It was one of many dreams I've had, especially after my disastrous online dating and in-person dating service experiences, one of of which, I described earlier. When you Google the topic of this chapter, Karine's website is the first that pops up. And here's why she says on her website why it works... even at this early stage of her business:

"This isn't your typical speed dating. We are committed to vegans and vegetarians. Our team is made up of longtime, active members of the veg community, and we spend all our energy figuring out how to find matches for veg singles only. Everyone you meet at our events will be vegan or vegetarian. We only partner with veg-friendly businesses and venues. And we definitely won't suggest you go *hunting* as a fun activity for your second date (yes, seriously, there is another site recommending that).

We Get the Details Right. Our events are set up for your success. Typically there will be 20-30 participants. For our heterosexual events, that means about 10-15 women and 10-15 men. In our 5+ years experience, this size is the most fun and optimises your chances of a real love match."

I can't stress the importance of finding a vegan soul mate, if that is where, in your deepest of deep thoughts, your heart is headed. As I've mentioned earlier, the traditional in-person dating services or speed dating meetings often don't go there. The testimonials on Veg Speed Date speak for themselves. It's as if the toughest and first layer of the onion is peeled back and you can fine tune the relationship goals and desires. I spent several months paying top dollar to go out with interesting men, but always feeling like they just didn't and would probably never get why I felt the way I did about my veganism. Veg Speed Date travels around the US, so look for them on their website at a city near you.

Online dating services have been around for a long time, with varying degrees of success. There's nothing quite like meeting a real person in real life, versus meeting them in real life after a bait and switch with a 30 year-old photo that looks nothing like current reality. As one of my dates who had had it with online services said, 'Did they not think I would ever meet the real person?"

With that caveat, along with the understanding that we all know you can be very creative with online profiles and the degree of truth they may hold, here are some options if you're shoppin.'

Other real life options are Meetups. You might feel intimidated at first, walking into a crowded restaurant or someone's home not knowing anyone. But it is well worth it. They're usually free and often are in potluck style, so you have the ability to taste many vegan options that you might never have imagined. Often, the meetup will request that the recipe be included with every dish so that you know what exactly is in the dish, and if there is anything that might be a sensitivity. Some people are squeamish about food someone else prepares, vegan or not, outside of a health department regulated restaurant. No worries. Bring your own and you know what you're eating, or just wait until you get back home to eat in your comfort zone. You won't starve for a few hours.

Just to give you an idea, Northwest Veg, which organizes the Portland Vegfest and many other things, lists 6 vegan meetup sites on their website, and five other vegan meetups in the Washington and Oregon areas. A part of the website lists physical buildings and businesses where you could hang out. Again, Portland being Portland, it has a vegan business district that takes up a full city block including the magical hangout of "Herbivore," which has SO many vegan shirts, you'll need to add an extra drawer or closet when you get home.

Of course, Portland is vegan mecca. But one could make that argument for almost any other city and state in the U.S. Just to give you an idea and some perspective, I first started speaking at vegfests in the US in 2011. The usual schedule was 1 or 2 a month. Now it is not unusual to find 2, and sometimes even 3 vegfests in the US on the same weekend. Those are great places to hang out with like-minded souls, too. But my main point is that the frequency of vegfests piling on top of each other now, is a testimonial to the wildly growing popularity of these events. Almost every vegfest I've spoken at has busted attendance numbers at the scene and has to move to a larger venue or use more space at that original venue. Some cities like Raleigh can even support two vegfests. Orlando has a vegfest and an Earth Day, organized by the same organizer with both events being vegan including the strict enforcement of vegan vendors. No exceptions. And the vegan police (you can even get a shirt with this printed on it) are out in force. Joking. ;) There is even a group in the Tampa Area, Solutionary Species, which has plans to organize as many vegfests as possible in the huge state of Florida. Most cities have a healthy selection of vegan restaurants. Spending an evening hanging out in a bar at a vegan restaurant is not the scourge that a typical bar scene might conjure up. I've had the pleasure of eating at many fine restaurants on book tour, especially with my publisher. Some of the classiest bars are at raw restaurants such as Cider Press Cafe in St. Petersburg, FL, where a single woman should have no problem checking out the local fare, food and otherwise. Check out Yelp or Happy Cow for restaurants in your area. In Florida alone, there are 428 restaurants listed. That's a lot to pick from, and not all in the largest cities. In Tampa, Florida Voices for Animals plans the area vegfest, but they also have a slew of events throughout the year. There's nothing like falling in love with a fellow protester who's been getting honked at all day long at the busiest shopping mall in town which has stores that sell fur.

If you are relegated to finding soulmates online, here are some options. Again the caveat: these lists are always changing and evolving. Please Google "resources for vegan singles and couples," and you'll get some local and distant options.

Planet Earth Singles: Nothing on the cover page about a vegan screen, just finding peace and bliss with a potential partner who shares candlelight dinners mainly to save money and be green.

Elite Singles is another online dating service but does not exclusively cater to vegans or vegetarians. However, they recognize the importance of being on the same page at the table saying, "Eating together is a huge part of dating and we understand the significance of sharing this experience with your partner. That's why we want to match you with fellow vegan singles."

There are the old stand-bys such as veggiedate, veggieconnection, vegandating.org, myveggetariandating.com, vegetariandatingservice.com, vegetarianpassions.com, greensingles.com and even an app for the busiest of the busiest, "Veg" that allows you to hook up on the run. Match.com claims it has the largest database of veggies, but who is going to verify that?

CHAPTER 15

Vegan Sex Toys and Products–Being Mission Consistent

At first, I thought how much could there be to this topic? And then I got blown away by stopping at a sex toy store on the way home from placing first in my age group at a 10K. It was a gorgeous Florida spring morning, and my lover and I were having a calm recovery breakfast at a large, popular restaurant, when we almost lost our vegan cookies.

A large truck, smaller than semi or so it seemed, pulled out of the parking lot onto the main road. A painting on the side of the truck, from one end to the other, advertised a sex toy store in rather graphic illustration which got everyone's attention. I immediately Googled it and much to our delight, we found we were only 8 minutes away. We quickly paid our bill and let GPS guide us to the very interesting store. The truck was parked on the parking lot, and I was surprised how much smaller it was when I got up close. Perhaps it was my wide-eyed stare that the graphics on the truck that made it seem larger than real life.

Neither my lover nor I had been to such a store together, and I think we were both believing we might find something we couldn't do without. My lover came to veganism through me, for health, and had only recently begun to get in touch with the animal welfare problems that are so pervasive around the globe. It seems like you can't go anywhere to escape. We were horrified to see so many sex toys that had real animal fur.

The saleswoman was quite enthusiastic, and I put on my investigative reporter's hat and played totally dumb. I asked her to show me everything, feigning delight and enthusiasm myself. I asked if I could take photos, mainly to help me remember all that I saw. I had no idea that vegan sex toys needs to be such a thing. I asked about fur, and she said, "Oh I know. I hate this," she said showing me hunks of animal fur hanging in strips from the wall. "Most of these kinds of things are from China. They're the worst offenders. (It is estimated that China makes 70% of the world's sex toys.) There's no regulation. I'm such an animal lover and I hate to see all this." Yeah, right. Kind of like someone at the local humane society who says, "I love animals," and then turns around and eats a hamburger for lunch. The disconnect is alive and well. She did show me one novelty from the popular company, Pipedream, which was clearly labeled, even though it was from China, metal and faux fur. Some people now have nickel allergies, and you can also find products labeled "nickel free."

As with any product you eat or wear, reading labels is critical. A tiny package of oral sex candy, a serving of 1, or about half an ounce, has a very high Amazon ranking at only $6. Such a bargain! Sold in the US, it does have the required nutrition facts label, which as you can imagine, is not rich in nutrition. The ingredients, listed in order of their quantities from the most to the least are: Sugar, corn syrup, citric acid, lactic acid, lactose and red dye #40. Not vegan. Not healthy. Mostly sugar. Yes, it is definitely correctly labeled as candy.

The employee almost embarrassed now, showed me several "bunny ears" that were made from real bunnies. Assorted feather boas and other body part decorations such as nipple covers included feathers too. The saleswoman gloated about how pleasure owners of these gadgets can now generate their own set of functions, or use memory control so that the product does exactly what they want, exactly how they like it, as soon as they turn it on. She showed a slew of vibrators and dildos that had multiple attachments, could move different ways, different speeds, rhythms and gyrations. She did a live demo of Bluetooth devices (well she didn't do an actual, precise demo, just a hypothetical one), which can improve the experience of teledildonics. Right. Those are high-tech sex toys that allow users to physically stimulate one another remotely. "Why yes," she said, "lovers can give each other a hard on and even orgasms by the remote controls on your phone's apps." Dildos now come with apps, giving new meaning to the trite phrase, "there's an app for that." Wireless Bullet had to be one of the more catchy names. Or the rechargeable, discreet, petite, powerful "Joie G-spot Stimulator." Forget your rechargeable plug? Some have USB cables if you can't upgrade to wireless. I came away from that whole sales presentation thinking that if things didn't work out with my real life lover, I could achieve an orgasm by plastics, silicone and remote control. Oh modern day technology! Seriously. Who needs a man?

I asked the saleswoman about the large truck. "Do you do in-home parties," I giggled. She giggled back. "No, I wish." No multi-level-marketing business model? No Tupperware or Fuckerware parties as my love cleverly chimed in the latter? "No," she said again. "The truck is strictly for picking up our merchandise and advertising around town." Pretty cool marketing plan driving that moving billboard all around town on a Saturday morning, stopping at the largest restaurant in town where people can't help but gawk. I wondered how many others followed their GPS for the same reason we did.

When I got back home, I started digging and was amazed to find this: A Forbes Magazine headline, "How The 'Niche' Sex Toy Market Grew Into An

Unstoppable $15B Industry" saying that the sex toys business has projections that it will surpass $50 billion by 2020. Just how much of that money is made off the backs of animals? That's a hard number to research. Some toys look like they're made with animal skins and fur and they're not. Other toys look like they are fakes but they're not.

I could easily envision animal activists expanding their protesting from puppy mills, circuses and animal captivity venues to sex toy stores. It was difficult for me to judge from the one store I visited how many products were made from animals. Most of the clothing that historically had been leather was a synthetic. It was easy to tell by reading the labels which clearly said, "all man made materials." Assuming the labels were true, of course. I think for the most part, if you touch the material, you can tell if it is from the skin of an animal. If there is any good news, there were far more products that weren't leather. The reason for that is, similar to the fading of leather shoes at some stores because manmade materials became far cheaper, so it goes with the kinky leather tight shirts, tops, straps and any other wearables and props that captured buyers. Simply, the faux leather is way cheaper now.

Feathers are quite another story. Original peacock feathers, often used in nipple covers or pasties, are pretty easy to spot with their vivid and intense colors. But other feathers, not so much. The store employee told me they had quite a few products with real feathers too. Fur, natural and artificially colored fur was used for bunny ear headbands and handcuffs.

Whether you want to be sticking silicone and pvc plastic up your vagina is your call. But if you don't, there is quite a variety of "organic," that's right, products you can choose from. You may be a persnickety shopper at Whole Foods, and you may be insistent that your investments are mission consistent by not having companies in your portfolio that test on animals. But are you equally particular when it comes to the bottom orifices? Shoppers don't often consider some of the nasty ingredients which are loaded into dildos, vibrators and dream cream lubricants. They largely go unregulated, even the products known as edibles. For my money, inserting or placing dates, grapes and berries in strategic locations, as long as you have towels to catch the juices, is a much safer and cheaper way to go. To see the USDA "organic" label on chamomile lubricant may be reassuring. Some lubricants actually have silicone in them. You may have to search for a vegan and chemical free lubricant. They do exist with labels such as "fusion of water and coconut oil." Which raises the question, why would you pay $24 for a 16 ounce can of that, when you could buy a whole lot of water and organic coconut oil for a lot less. It may be hard to pass by the neon silicone slim dongs, though. They come in all sizes, shapes and colors. We are not vegan virgins anymore, are we?

One of the biggest problems for the industry is the popularity of toys that are made from PVC, or polyvinyl chlorides. Think PVC plumbing pipes. But those wouldn't feel so good, so the industry softened the plastic with another controversial chemical, phthalates. These plastics are cheap and easy to work with. However, studies have shown that exposure to phthalates can cause cancer. Minute levels have been linked to sperm damage. A German study in 2000 found 10 dangerous chemicals off-gassed in some sex toys in Europe, although the store saleswoman assured that the Europeans, long known for their strict food controls, have the strictest controls on their sex toys. Part of the problem is the long shelf life of these products, whether sitting out on a store shelf or a consumer's shelf. Some of the products deteriorate over time, and if they come into contact with fat, it helps draw the phthalates out of the plastic. Not good for a warm, moist vagina. Interestingly, children's toys are regulated in the US by the Consumer Product Safety Commission. The US, Europe, Canada and Japan have tight controls keeping phthalates out of children's toys and bodies, but not so much for adults. The packaging of sex toys is often labeled as a "novelty," which allows it to scoot under the radar.

Some companies have taken matters into their own hands simply by not offering products with phthalate. Others recommend using a condom with a toy.

Other stores, such as Smitten Kitten, chose when they began business not to carry jellies, cyberskins or any other questionable toy. Getting a good reputation from the start was important.

Wait. Let's go back a sentence. As I was researching, I assumed that cyberskin meant a covering on a toy that feels like a smartphone's silky, silicone or "skin" covering. But then, I found it on Amazon. You can too. For $175. It's not just a toy. It's an anatomically correct toy, called the "vibrating perfect butt." For those of you who have always wanted a perfect butt, there you go. And without the hassle of a relationship. Vegan lubricants sold separately. There's hardly a day that doesn't go by researching for this book when I don't feel like a babe in the woods, a virgin almost, when it comes to the incredible diversity of choices in the sex toy world. Who knew? I certainly did not.

If you don't want to play with fire, there's always the almost reliable standby. The safest sex is practiced with condoms, but not all condoms are vegan. In fact, most aren't. Some are even made using casein, a form of cow's milk protein. Others are made from lamb intestines. Major ewwww…

Vegan condoms include Sustain, Glyde, Sir Richard's Condom Company and Durex, which includes non-latex condoms for those who have sensitivities. Only a few of their lines are vegan. They include: Ultra, Deluxe, Featherlite and Avanti Ultima. Fair-Squared is lubricated vegan condom. Who knew? How many times have you said this reading along? I know I did almost every time I Googled. FC2 Internal Condoms says on its website:

"Get hot and steamy with the pre-lubricated FC2 Female Condom. It warms to your body temperature so you'll feel the heat during intimacy! It's easy to use and can enhance your pleasure and your partner's pleasure too! Latex free and body safe."

These are nitrile condoms and are intended to be worn inside the vagina or anus. In case you're wondering what nitrile is made of, because so often, replacements for bad chemicals are worse, nitrile rubber is also known as

Buna-N, Perbunan, acrylonitrile butadiene rubber, and NBR, is a synthetic rubber copolymer of acrylonitrile (ACN) and butadiene. Trade names include Nipol, Krynac and Europrene. If you know what all those names mean, you must be a chemist. I just copied the definition from Wiki.

Vegan lubricants include Good Clean Love's Almost Naked Personal Lubricant. And who, better to launch TheVeganSexShop.com but a winner of PETA's 2007 Sexiest Vegetarian Next Door? The store has condoms, candles, and all kinds of sex toys. The owner makes the point that it's important to be able to trust that every product is 100% cruelty-free, and in an ideal world, buyers are supporting a vegan business.

Once again, this topic is on fire online. Many blogs and websites list fav vegan sex toy stores. Google, of course, for a current listing. There are way too many vegan sex toy websites to mention. Overwhelming, in fact. So many creative website names. Afemmecock has one of the most extensive listings of any online source for your prurient interests. Some websites even go into great detail about the various categories of sex toys. Oh, just take a look in the retailer category:

Retailers

Safe Sex Barriers

Lube

Strap-On Harnesses

Impact Toys

Bondage

Collars and Body Harnesses

Gags

Other Good Stuff

A word or 2 needs to be said on behalf of feminist vegan agitators, and others who care about the objectification of women that seems to be growing in a world that seems to care less about all animals. I often say, I'm just the reporter. Don't kill the messenger. Personally, I'm not into bondage, collars, BDSM or any other behaviors that exploit women or men. Even in fantasy. The point of the above is to show you that just because someone is vegan, or has a vegan business, doesn't mean it aligns with your values. Further, as stated, the sex toys business is huge and covers a wide range of interests, that used to be considered over the top. But ever since Bill Clinton and popular programs such as "Sex in the City," and movies like "50 Shades of Grey" have taken some of our most deviant fantasies out of the box, the sex toys business has exploded. This is not just my opinion, but that of the store owners and the articles that have been written about them.

As a young TV reporter in St. Louis, I remember the case of a woman who's hanging body was found burned in her garage. Her boyfriend had engaged in some sex game with a noose around the neck, creating oxygen deprivation which supposedly enhanced the woman's orgasm. Obviously it didn't go so well when she died. He set the garage on fire to cover the evidence. Like the botched sex act, that didn't go so well either. Our assignment editor became obsessed with the case and eventually wrote a book about it called, "Dying to Get Married." As a result of that and other similar, though perhaps not as much of a fatal attraction as death by orgasm, there is a segment of the population that not only finds this kind of behavior or fantasy as pretty revolting and not worthy of a single additional thought. However, many people do go there, and it is just the way it is. To that end, I come full circle, connecting the dots by saying, if you're going to buy the bondage toys, harnesses and collars, please, go vegan. For the sake of your health, the planet, the animals, and your partner.

Some of the more popular vegan sex toy stores online are: Ethical Kink, The Sensual Vegan, Goodkink, and Justine and Julliette.

I hope what we've written becomes a good resource based on your interests. However, I reach the end of my writing and feel like I did when I got the name as a financial consultant, based on my organic gardening and staying at home 6 years to breastfeed my 3 daughters, "Earth Mother in a Suit." With all this information, I just want to run back under the covers with my lover and do it similar to the Smith Barney ad that was so popular… "the old fashioned way." Hey, if it ain't broke, don't fix it. If your vegan sex is going well and making all your parts and your significant other's part hum right along, that can be fine enough. At least, for the most part, you know what you're getting and what's coming. Last and final pun. Have fun out there! We are definitely no longer vegan virgins.

Vegan Sex Recipes

The larger the vegan movement, if we may call it that, grows, the more we encompass different opinions. There is no larger controversy in the vegan universe on whether to eat/add fat or not. The low-fat plant-based doctors say if you are trying to avoid heart disease, and especially if you already have beginning or full-blown heart disease, based on research, you should avoid added fats and oils. Other doctors are not so quick to swear off nuts and seeds, and their processed oils, understanding that in the grand scheme of things, if a person is healthy, a tablespoon of nuts or oil once in awhile is not going to result in an instant heart attack. Oils are considered a processed food and run the risk of going rancid from oxidation in just a few months, depending on storage.

Especially if it means the difference between remaining vegan long-term or not, some pundits encourage using some omega 3 and 6 healthy fats such as avocados and flaxseed oil. These fat sources can be good for the brain, but if you are concerned, it is always a good idea to get baseline blood tests to make sure everything is OK. Vegan athletes often include a diet rich in nuts and seeds, as much for calories and feeling satisfied as anything.

Sometimes I feel, and I've heard other women agree, that looking at a nut makes us gain weight. Nuts are indeed, very calorie dense and should be the first to cut back on or even go if you are seriously overweight trying to dump some body fat.

The general guideline I use is, "What did Mother Nature intended?" and "How did our ancestors really eat?" I doubt any of our ancient ancestors were stomping on olives trying to squeeze out the oil. This major disagreement in our community won't go away soon. In the recipes below, if you want to reduce the oils or added fats, knock yourself out, though understand that it might change the recipe outcome. If you are OK with adding the fats suggested in the recipes that include them, go for it. The other option of course, is to omit these recipes and use others. This is such a hot button issue, we have tried to walk the diplomatic and scientific fences as best we can.

It seems that many things are controversial these days, and one more area that has generated controversy is cast iron cookware which Beverly offers as an option in some recipes. A little iron can be good for a vegan who need this important mineral. But in some cases, it doesn't take too much iron absorption to create problems. When in doubt, use a different skillet.

CHAPTER 16

Morning Quickies–Quick Beverages and Morning Options

We all lead busy lives and have to juggle many things. Getting moving in the morning can be a real struggle for some, and we often find ourselves running short on time and in need of a quick fix for fueling our bodies. Maybe you're one of those people who have trouble getting their kids or themselves up and at 'em? Or if you're lucky, maybe you actually "got in a morning quickie" and that's what made you run late...hmm? Whatever the case, the quick and easy beverages, smoothies, fruit-based bowls, and breakfast spreads and sandwich recipes in this chapter will help get your day off to a great start!

Chai Tea for Two

MAKES 2 SERVINGS

India is famous for its delicious and comforting chai tea. Chai is made by brewing black tea with an aromatic blend of warmth-enhancing spices, such as cardamom, cinnamon, cloves, ginger, and pepper or nutmeg, and then the flavorful tea is blended with milk and lightly sweetened. Check the tea section of your local grocery or natural foods store for a prepackaged chai tea blend.

- 1½ cups water
- 2 chai tea bags
- 1 cup almond milk, coconut milk beverage, or other nondairy milk
- 1½ tablespoons coconut sugar, agave nectar, or other sweetener
- 1 teaspoon vanilla extract

1. Put the water and tea bags in a small saucepan. Bring to a boil over high heat. Remove from the heat. Let the tea steep for 5 minutes. Remove and discard the tea bags.

2. While the tea is steeping, put the milk and sugar in a medium saucepan and cook over medium heat, stirring occasionally, until hot and bubbles appear on the surface.

3. Remove from the heat. Stir in the vanilla extract. Add the chai tea and whisk until frothy. Evenly divide mixture between two glasses. Serve immediately.

Iced Chai Latté: Allow the finished chai tea mixture to cool completely, and then pour over ice cubes to serve.

Mango Lassi

MAKES 2 SERVINGS

Lassi beverages come in a wide assortment of fruity flavors and are commonly served in Indian restaurants to provide a cooling effect when eating curries and other spicy dishes. This lightly sweetened, creamy, and refreshing drink is made with non dairy yogurt, juicy mango, and aromatic cardamom and rose water.

- 1½ cups nondairy milk
- 1 mango, peeled, pitted, and diced
- 1 container (6 ounces) plain or vanilla nondairy yogurt
- 1 tablespoon agave nectar or coconut sugar, or 2 pitted soft dates (preferably medjool dates)
- 1 teaspoon rose water (optional)
- ½ teaspoon ground cardamom
- Ice cubes (optional)

1. Put all of the ingredients in a blender and process until smooth. Scrape down the sides of the container with a spatula and process for 15 seconds.

2. Evenly divide mixture between two glasses. Serve immediately, as is or over ice cubes as desired.

Variation: For an extra creamy version, prepare with coconut milk beverage. Also, individual servings can be garnished with finely chopped pistachios or almonds as desired.

Arousing Avocado Green Smoothie

MAKES 2 SERVINGS

Make this green smoothie for the man in your life to help boost his libido. It contains many fruits and veggies that are reminiscent of male anatomy, such as dates, banana, cucumber, celery, and avocado (which the Aztecs affectionately called a "testicle tree," as the fruit hangs in pairs), along with some stamina-enhancing chia seeds.

- 2 cups baby spinach, kale, or other leafy greens, stemmed and lightly packed
- 1 cup coconut water or water
- 1 banana, broken into 4 pieces
- 1 avocado, diced
- ⅔ cup diced cucumber
- 1 large stalk celery, sliced
- ½ cup ice cubes
- ¼ cup fresh mint or basil leaves, lightly packed
- 3 pitted soft dates
- Juice of ½ a lemon
- ¼ cup raw pistachios
- 2 teaspoons chia seeds

1. Put all of the ingredients in a blender and process until smooth. Scrape down the sides of the container with a spatula and process for 15 seconds.

2. Evenly divide mixture between two glasses. Serve immediately.

Variation: Replace the coconut water with 1 cup cold green tea for an energizing mid-morning or post-workout boost.

Hot Bahama Mama Smoothie
MAKES 2 SERVINGS

The inspiration for this smoothie comes from the popular rum-based cocktail known as a Bahama Mama. This non-alcoholic version is made with a variety of exotic fruits, coconut milk, orange juice, plus a little jalapeño chile and ginger for a zesty, tongue-tingling zing! This luscious smoothie captures the flavor of a tropical island paradise.

- 1½ cups fresh or frozen papaya chunks
- 1½ cups fresh, canned, or frozen pineapple chunks or pineapple tidbits
- 1 mango, peeled, pitted, and diced
- 1 cup plain or vanilla coconut milk beverage
- ½ cup fresh or frozen sweet or sour cherries, pitted, or ¼ cup pomegranate seeds
- Juice of 1 lime
- ½ a small jalapeño chile, seeded
- 1 (1-inch) piece fresh ginger, thinly sliced

1. Put all of the ingredients in a blender and process until smooth. Scrape down the sides of the container with a spatula and process for 15 seconds.

2. Evenly divide mixture between two glasses. Serve immediately.

Variation: Feel free to replace any of the suggested fruits with other exotic fruits, such as guava, dragon fruit, star fruit, or passion fruit. If you would like, you can add one or two shots of light rum or coconut rum.

Bahamas Breakfast Bowls: Using only ½ of the mango in the smoothie mixture. Evenly divide the smoothie mixture between two bowls. Top each serving with ½ of the remaining diced mango, ½ of a peeled, halved, and sliced kiwi, and 1 tablespoon of pomegranate seeds or goji berries. Serve immediately.

Dutch Apple Pie Smoothie

MAKES 2 SERVINGS

Apples, rolled oats, walnuts, flax seeds, and spices are blended to perfection, and one taste of this aphrodisiac-augmented smoothie will fool your taste buds into thinking that you're eating a slice of Dutch apple pie for breakfast.

- ⅔ cup old-fashioned rolled oats
- ¼ cup raw walnuts
- 2 teaspoons flaxseeds
- 1 cup water or coconut water
- 1 cup plain or vanilla almond milk or other nondairy milk
- 2 medium apples, cored and coarsely chopped
- 4 pitted soft dates
- 1½ teaspoons vanilla extract
- 1 teaspoon ground cinnamon
- ¼ teaspoon freshly grated nutmeg

1. Put the oats, walnuts, and flaxseeds in a blender and process into a fine flour, about 30 seconds.

2. Add the water, milk, apples, dates, vanilla extract, cinnamon, and nutmeg and process until smooth. Scrape down the sides of the container with a spatula and process for 15 seconds.

3. Evenly divide mixture between two glasses. Serve immediately.

Mexican Hot Chocolate Smoothie

MAKES 2 SERVINGS

The Mayan and Aztec Indians of Mexico were among the first civilizations to cultivate cacao trees and to enjoy chocolate-flavored beverages. This hot chocolate-inspired smoothie is enhanced with vanilla, cinnamon, and cayenne, and a few sips will surely warm you from the inside out.

- 2 cups plain, vanilla, or chocolate almond milk or other nondairy milk
- ½ cup ice cubes, or ½ of a banana, peeled and broken in half
- 3 tablespoons cacao powder or unsweetened cocoa powder
- 2 tablespoons light brown sugar or coconut sugar
- 1 teaspoon vanilla extract
- ¾ teaspoon ground cinnamon
- ⅛ teaspoon cayenne or chili powder

1. Put all of the ingredients in a blender and process until smooth. Scrape down the sides of the container with a spatula and process for 15 seconds.

2. Evenly divide mixture between two glasses. Serve immediately.

Maca-Mochaccino Smoothie: Replace 1 cup of the almond milk with 1 cup cold coffee. Use only ¼ teaspoon ground cinnamon. Replace the cayenne with 2 tablespoons maca powder.

Ambrosia

MAKES 2 SERVINGS

According to Greek mythology, ambrosia was the food of the gods, which, if eaten regularly, would bestow immortality and longevity onto the gods and humans that consumed it. For those of you who prefer a light morning meal, this refreshing fruit salad is ideal, as it's made of oranges, pineapple, banana, pomegranate seeds, and shredded coconut.

- 2 oranges, or 1 navel and 1 blood orange, peeled
- 1 banana, cut into 1-inch slices
- ½ cup fresh, canned, or frozen (thawed) pineapple chunks or pineapple tidbits
- 1 tablespoon agave nectar
- ¼ cup pomegranate seeds
- 2 tablespoons unsweetened shredded dried coconut

1. Cut the oranges into segments, over a medium bowl to catch the juices, and dropping the segments into the bowl.

2. Add the banana, pineapple, and agave nectar and stir to combine. Scatter the pomegranate seeds and shredded coconut over the top. Serve immediately.

Passion Fruit Breakfast Bowls

MAKES 2 SERVINGS

Smoothie bowls are all the rage! Rather than sipping, bowlfuls of the smoothie mixture are topped with additional ingredients, like dried or chopped fruits, and eaten with a spoon. What's more, you'll get your partner in a relaxed mood in the morning by serving them some passion fruit, which is known for its exotic flavor and sedative-like properties.

- 1 mango, peeled, pitted, and diced
- 1 cup fresh, canned, or frozen pineapple chunks or pineapple tidbits
- 1 frozen banana, broken into 4 pieces
- ½ cup coconut water or plain nondairy milk
- 1 passion fruit
- 1 kiwi, peeled, cut into quarters lengthwise, and thinly sliced
- 2 tablespoons goji berries

1. Put ½ of the mango, pineapple, banana, and coconut water in a blender and process until smooth. Scrape down the sides of the container with a spatula and process for 15 seconds.

2. Evenly divide the blended mixture between two bowls. Cut the passion fruit in half, scoop half of the seeds into each bowl, and then stir the seeds into the mixture in a swirl pattern.

3. Top each serving with ½ of the remaining diced mango, ½ a sliced kiwi, and 1 tablespoon of goji berries. Serve immediately.

Pistachio, Dried Fruit, and Yogurt Delight
MAKES 2 SERVINGS

The creamy, yogurt-based Shrikhand is a popular treat in India. For this version, saffron threads and ground cardamom are pulverized with powdered sugar, which both tints and flavors the yogurt. For a final flourish, the flavored yogurt is blended and garnished with chopped figs and dates, as well as crunchy pistachios.

- ¼ cup powdered sugar or coconut sugar
- ½ teaspoon saffron threads
- ⅛ teaspoon ground cardamom
- 2 containers (6 ounces) or ⅔ cup plain or vanilla nondairy yogurt
- ½ teaspoon rose water (optional)
- ⅓ cup raw pistachios, coarsely chopped
- 4 dried figs, coarsely chopped
- 4 pitted soft dates, coarsely chopped

1. Put the powdered sugar, saffron threads, and cardamom in a food processor or blender and process for 30 to 60 seconds, until the saffron is finely ground.

2. Put the yogurt in a medium bowl. Add the sugar mixture and optional rose water and stir to combine.

3. Add ½ of the chopped pistachios, figs, and dates and stir to combine.

4. Cover and refrigerate for 30 minutes or more, before serving, to allow the flavors to blend. Scatter the remaining chopped pistachios, figs, and dates over the top and serve.

Good Morning Muesli

MAKES 2 SERVINGS

For an effortless yet filling breakfast, muesli is the answer. This old-fashioned and ever-popular Swiss breakfast offering can best be described as a cross between a porridge and granola. For this recipe, rolled oats are softened simply by soaking them overnight in the refrigerator in some nondairy milk and yogurt. In the morning, the softened oats are combined with a few other ingredients to create a creamy breakfast cereal.

- 1 cup old-fashioned rolled oats
- 1 cup plain or vanilla nondairy milk
- 2 containers (6 ounces) or ⅔ cup plain or vanilla nondairy yogurt
- 2 teaspoons ground flaxseeds or flaxseed meal
- 1 large apple, coarsely chopped
- ¼ cup nuts (such as almonds, pecans, or walnuts), coarsely chopped
- 2 tablespoons raisins, or 1 tablespoon dried currants
- 2 tablespoons dried cranberries or cherries
- Ground cinnamon
- Maple syrup

1. Put the rolled oats, milk, yogurt, and flaxseeds in a medium bowl and stir to combine. Cover and refrigerate overnight.

2. Stir the oat mixture. Add the apple, nuts, raisins, and cranberries and stir to combine.

3. Evenly divide the oat mixture between two bowls. Top each serving with cinnamon and maple syrup as desired. Serve immediately.

Grab Bag Granola

MAKES 4 CUPS OR 8 (½ CUP) SERVINGS

Sure you can buy pre-made granola from a store, but they often contain excessive amounts of sweeteners, salt, and oil. When you make it yourself, then you get to control what's in it, as well as the final flavor. Also, the baking granola will fill your house with a tantalizing aroma. Enjoy bowlfuls of this granola as a cold cereal with nondairy milk, or eat it by the handful as an after sex snack.

- 2 cups old-fashioned rolled oats or other whole grain flakes (such as barley, spelt, or triticale)
- ½ cup oat bran or wheat bran
- ½ cup raw sliced almonds
- ½ cup raw sunflower seeds
- ¼ cup ground flaxseeds or flaxseed meal
- ¾ teaspoon ground cinnamon
- ¾ teaspoon ground fenugreek
- ⅛ teaspoon ground nutmeg
- ¼ cup coconut water or apple juice
- 2 tablespoons maple syrup
- 2 tablespoons sunflower oil or other oil
- ½ teaspoon almond extract
- ½ teaspoon vanilla extract
- ½ cup dried fruit (such as raisins, cherries, cranberries, currants, chopped dates, chopped apricots, or a combination)

1. Preheat the oven to 325 degrees F. Line a baking sheet with parchment paper or a silicone baking mat.

2. Put the rolled oats, oat bran, almonds, sunflower seeds, flaxseeds, cinnamon, fenugreek, and nutmeg in a large bowl and stir to combine.

3. Put the coconut water, maple syrup, oil, almond extract, and vanilla extract in a small bowl and whisk to combine. Pour the coconut mixture over the oat mixture and stir to combine.

4. Transfer the oat mixture to the lined baking sheet and spread into a single layer with a spatula.

5.   Bake for 20 minutes. Remove from the oven. Stir with a metal spatula
     and spread into a single layer again. Bake for 20 to 25 minutes longer,
     until golden brown and dry.

6.   Sprinkle the dried fruit over the top and stir until evenly distributed. Let
     cool completely. Store in an airtight container at room temperature.

Strawberry-Cashew Cream Cheese Spread

MAKES 2 CUPS OR 8 (¼ CUP) SERVINGS

Homemade cashew cream cheese is combined with juicy strawberries to create this luscious and slightly sweet spread. This tasty spread is a great topping for toast or bagels, as well as a dip for sliced fresh fruit or celery sticks.

- 1 cup sliced strawberries
- ¼ cup powdered sugar, coconut sugar, or agave nectar
- 1½ teaspoons vanilla extract
- 1 cup raw cashews (soaked for 1 hour or more and drained)
- ¼ cup water or coconut water
- 1 tablespoon nutritional yeast flakes
- 1 tablespoon lemon juice
- Pinch of sea salt

1. Put the strawberries, sugar, and vanilla extract in a small bowl and stir to combine. Let sit for 5 minutes to macerate.

2. Put the cashews, water, nutritional yeast, lemon juice, and a pinch of salt in a food processor and process until smooth. Scrape down the sides of the container with a spatula and process for 15 seconds.

3. Add the strawberry mixture and process until smooth. Transfer the mixture to an airtight container and refrigerate for 30 minutes or more, before serving, to allow the flavors to blend.

Herbed-Cashew Cream Cheese Spread: Omit the strawberries, powdered sugar, and vanilla extract. When blending the cashew mixture, add an additional 3 tablespoons water and 1 tablespoon nutritional yeast flakes, ½ teaspoon onion powder, and½ teaspoon garlic powder. Transfer to an airtight container, and stir in 2 tablespoon chopped fresh basil or parsley, and 1 thinly sliced green onion or 2 finely chopped chives.

Avocado Toast with Coconut Bacon

MAKES 2 SERVINGS

Slightly sweet and smoky coconut bacon has become a life-changer for vegans who miss the taste of bacon, and it's quite easy to make in your oven. For this recipe, the crispy morsels are used as a topping for slices of toast that have been slathered with mashed avocado, and one bite is sure to rock your world!

Coconut bacon:
- ¾ teaspoon maple syrup
- ½ teaspoon reduced-sodium tamari or coconut aminos
- ¼ teaspoon chili powder or smoked or sweet paprika
- ½ cup unsweetened coconut chips

- 1 avocado, diced
- Juice of ½ a lemon
- Sea salt
- Crushed red pepper flakes
- 2 slices whole grain bread or other bread of choice, toasted

1. To make the coconut bacon, preheat the oven to 325 degrees F. Line a baking sheet with parchment paper or a silicone baking mat.

2. Put the maple syrup, tamari, and chili powder in a small bowl and stir to combine. Add the coconut chips and stir to evenly coat the coconut chips with the mixture.

3. Transfer the coconut mixture to the lined baking sheet and spread into a single layer with a spatula. Bake for 10 to 12 minutes, stirring every 5 minutes, until the coconut chips are golden brown. Watch closely during the last 2 minutes of baking time, to avoid burning it.

4. Remove from the oven. Let cool completely. The coconut bacon will become crispier as it cools.

5. To make the avocado toast, put the avocado and lemon juice in a small bowl and mash with a fork until desired consistency. Season with salt and red pepper flakes to taste.

6. Evenly dividing, spread the avocado mixture on the toasted bread slices, and then top with the coconut bacon as desired. Serve immediately.

Variation: You can use the coconut bacon as a topping for soups, salads, sandwiches, and sides and main dishes.

Avocado Toast with Tomato: If you're short on time, forego making the coconut bacon. Instead top the avocado mixture on each piece of toast with 2 tablespoons diced tomatoes.

Fruit-n-Nut Rice Cakes

MAKES 2 SERVINGS

Your taste buds will be delighted and surprised by the juxtaposition of the tart goji berries with the sweet bananas and cinnamon, which are served atop a nut butter-covered rice cake. This open-faced sandwich is nutritious and delicious, and makes for a great snack or on-the-go breakfast when you're short on time.

- 2 rice cakes (variety of choice)
- 2 tablespoons nut butter (such as almond, cashew, or peanut butter)
- 1 tablespoon raw sunflower seeds
- 1 tablespoon goji berries, raisins, or dried cranberries
- Ground cinnamon
- 1 medium banana, thinly sliced

1. Place each rice cake on a plate. Evenly spread 1 tablespoon of nut butter over the top of each rice cake.

2. Scatter 1½ teaspoons of sunflower seeds and goji berries over the top of each rice cake, and then gently press them into the nut butter with your fingers. Sprinkle cinnamon over the top as desired. Evenly dividing, top each with banana slices. Serve immediately.

CHAPTER 17

Lingering Breakfasts
(or Brunches) in Bed–Breakfast/Brunch Options and Baked Goods

Breakfast really is the most important meal of the day. After all, you're breaking your overnight fast of not eating for up to 8 hours or more--unless you ate after your late-night booty call! So, it really makes sense to eat something substantial for your first meal of the day. The recipes in this chapter are great for breakfast or brunch, as they're a little more involved than the ones in the previous chapter. Therefore, they do take a little more time to prepare, and they're better suited for when you've got plenty of time to cook, like on the weekend or when you're having a lazy day around the house. Ahead, you'll find veganized versions of classic breakfast items, like French toast, pancakes, bacon, sausages, and a scramble. For those who like to bake, you'll also find a biscuit, scone, banana bread, and muffin recipes as well.

Rum Banana Roll Ups

MAKES 2 SERVINGS

Make these breakfast roll ups when you feel like being a little bit naughty in the morning. A mixture of yogurt, dates, almonds, and coconut is used as part of the filling for flour tortillas, which tastes delicious on its own, but the rum-soaked banana topping is what's sure to make you swoon!

Rum bananas:
- 2 large bananas, cut into 1-inch thick slices
- ¼ cup coconut water or water
- 1 tablespoon agave nectar or maple syrup
- ½ teaspoon ground cinnamon
- 2 tablespoons rum (light, dark, or coconut rum)

Roll Ups:
- ½ cup plain or vanilla nondairy yogurt

- ¼ cup pitted soft dates, coarsely chopped
- ¼ cup raw or toasted sliced almonds
- 3 tablespoons unsweetened coconut chips, or 1 tablespoon unsweetened shredded dried coconut, toasted
- ½ teaspoon vanilla extract, or ¼ teaspoon almond extract
- 2 (8-inch or larger) flour tortillas

1. To make the rum bananas, put the bananas and coconut water in a large cast iron or nonstick skillet and cook over medium heat, stirring occasionally, for 2 minutes.

2. Add the agave nectar and cinnamon, decrease to low heat, and cook, stirring occasionally, for 2 minutes.

3. Add the rum and cook, stirring occasionally, for 1 minute, until bananas are soft. Alternatively, the banana mixture can be flambéed by carefully igniting the mixture and letting the alcohol burn off before serving (see Tips in Cherries Jubilee in Happy Endings).

4. To make the filling, put the yogurt, dates, almonds, coconut, and vanilla extract in a small bowl and stir to combine.

5. For easier rolling, warm each tortilla in a large skillet over medium heat, for 1 minute per side, or in a microwave oven for 20 to 30 seconds.

6. To assemble the roll ups, place each tortilla on a large plate. Spoon half of the yogurt mixture in the center of each tortilla. Top with one-quarter of the rum bananas (just the banana slices). Fold the bottom of the tortilla over the filling and continue rolling it over like a crêpe. Evenly dividing, spoon the remaining rum bananas mixture over the top of each roll up. Serve immediately.

Variation: If you're not in the mood for booze at breakfast, replace the rum with an additional 1 tablespoon agave nectar or maple syrup. Also, the rum bananas mixture can be used as a topping for nondairy ice cream, cake, or other desserts.

Vanilla-Almond French Toast

MAKES 2 SERVINGS OR 4 SLICES

Using your blender, you can quickly and easily bang out a vanilla and almond-enhanced batter, which will transform ordinary slices of bread into fabulous French toast. If you've got some maca powder, then add it to the mix, as it will rev up the flavor and your libido. Serve the French toast with your choice of toppings, like maple syrup, agave nectar, or jam.

• ⅔ cup water or coconut water	• 1 teaspoon ground flaxseeds or flaxseed meal
• ⅓ whole raw almonds	• 2 teaspoons vanilla extract
• 3 pitted soft dates (preferably medjool dates)	• ¼ teaspoon almond extract
• 1 tablespoon maca powder (optional)	• ¼ teaspoon sea salt
	• 4 slices whole grain bread or other bread of choice

1. Put all of the ingredients (except the bread slices) in a blender and process until smooth. Scrape down the sides of the container jar with a spatula and process for 15 seconds.

2. Transfer the mixture to 9 x13-inch baking pan. Place the bread slices in the baking pan and flip over each slice to evenly coat on all sides. Let the bread slices soak in the mixture for 1 minute.

3. Lightly oil a large cast iron or nonstick skillet or griddle, or mist it with cooking spray. Heat over medium heat.

4. When the skillet is hot, place the bread slices into it and cook, for 2 to 3 minutes, until golden brown on the bottom. You will need to cook the bread slices in several batches depending on the size of the skillet. Flip the bread slices over with a spatula and cook, for 2 to 3 minutes, until golden brown on the other side. Serve hot, 2 slices per person with your choice of toppings as desired.

Berry Nice and Spice Pancakes

MAKES 2 SERVINGS OR 4 PANCAKES

Forget going to the diner, and instead, make your lover a batch of these light and fluffy pancakes. The batter for these pancakes is flavored with vanilla, a bit of spice, and your favorite sweet and juicy berries. If you're feeling a bit adventurous, use a combination of berries. Serve them with your choice of toppings, like maple syrup, jam, or additional berries.

- 2 cups whole wheat flour or whole wheat pastry flour
- 1½ tablespoons aluminum-free baking powder
- 1 teaspoon ground cinnamon
- ½ teaspoon ground cardamom or ground ginger
- Pinch of sea salt
- 2 cups plain or vanilla nondairy milk
- 1 tablespoon maple syrup
- 1½ teaspoons vanilla extract
- 1 cup fresh or frozen berries (such as blackberries, blueberries, raspberries, sliced strawberries, or mixed berries)

1. Put the flour, baking powder, cinnamon, cardamom, and salt in a large bowl and whisk to combine.

2. Add the milk, maple syrup, and vanilla extract and whisk until just combined (a few lumps are fine, but don't over mix or the pancakes will be tough). Gently stir in the berries. Let the batter sit for 5 minutes.

3. Lightly oil a large cast iron or nonstick skillet, or griddle, or mist it with cooking spray. Heat over medium heat.

4. When the skillet is hot, pour the batter into it using ½ cup of batter for each pancake. You will need to cook the pancakes in several batches depending on the size of the skillet. Cook for 2 to 3 minutes, until the edges of the pancakes are slightly dry and bubbles appear on top. Flip the pancakes over with a spatula and cook for 2 to 3 minutes, until golden brown on the other side.

5. Lightly oil the skillet again and repeat the cooking procedure with the remaining batter. Serve hot, 2 pancakes per person with your choice of toppings as desired.

Variation: For gluten-free pancakes, replace the whole wheat flour with buckwheat flour. Or if you prefer, use a gluten-free baking blend, and also add ¾ teaspoon xanthan gum to the dry ingredients.

Baked Latkes with Applesauce

MAKES 4 SERVINGS (2 LATKES AND ¼ CUP APPLESAUCE PER SERVING)

Whether you call them potato latkes or potato pancakes, you're going to love these patties made from shredded potatoes, onion, and a few seasonings. Typically, potato latkes are pan-fried in oil, but this healthier version is made without any oil, and they're oven-baked instead. You can serve them with the suggested applesauce, or, if you prefer, enjoy them without it.

Applesauce:
- 2 medium apples, peeled, cored, and diced
- ½ cup apple juice or water

Latkes:
- 2 large Russet potatoes, peeled
- 1 small yellow onion
- ¼ cup chopped fresh parsley, lightly packed
- 2 tablespoons finely chopped chives, or ¼ cup thinly sliced green onions

- 3 tablespoons chickpea flour, whole wheat flour, or potato starch
- 1½ tablespoons nutritional yeast flakes
- 1 teaspoon garlic powder
- ½ teaspoon aluminum-free baking powder
- ½ teaspoon sea salt
- ¼ teaspoon freshly ground black pepper

1. To make the applesauce, put the apples and apple juice in a small saucepan. Bring to a boil over medium heat. Cover, decrease the heat to low, and simmer for 15 to 20 minutes, until the apples are tender. Remove from the heat and uncover the saucepan. Let cool for 10 minutes.

2. Using a potato masher or a fork, mash the apple mixture to desired consistency. Serve warm or cold as desired.

3. To make the potato latkes, preheat the oven to 425 degrees F. Line a baking sheet with parchment paper or a silicone baking liner.

4. Using a food processor or box grater, finely shred the potatoes and onion. Put the shredded potatoes and onion in a large bowl and cover with cold water (to prevent the potatoes from discoloring).

5. Using your hands, grab large handfuls of the potato-onion mixture, and squeeze out as much of the water as possible (as the drier they are the crispier the latkes will be). Place each squeezed-out handful of the potato-onion mixture into a medium bowl.

6. Stir with a fork to loosen up the shredded the potato-onion mixture. Add the remaining ingredients and stir to combine.

7. Using a ¼ cup measuring cup, portion each potato latke by lightly filling and gently packing the mixture into the cup with the back of a spoon. Flip the measuring cup over onto the lined baking sheet and tap the cup to release the mixture. Repeat the procedure with the remaining mixture. Slightly flatten each portion with your fingers.

8. Bake on the bottom oven rack for 15 minutes. Remove from the oven. Flip the potato latkes over with a metal spatula. Bake for 10 to 15 minutes longer, until golden brown on both sides. Serve hot. Top the potato latkes with applesauce as desired.

Tempeh Bacon

MAKES 4 SERVINGS OR 8 SLICES

Thin slices of tempeh are marinated in a blend of tamari, maple syrup, apple cider vinegar, toasted sesame oil, and some spices. Then the marinated slices are oven-baked until golden brown, and you'll go crazy over the flavor of these savory slices. Serve the tempeh bacon for breakfast, use them on sandwiches or salads, or add them to your favorite recipes.

- 2 tablespoons reduced-sodium tamari or coconut aminos
- 1 tablespoon maple syrup
- 1½ tablespoons apple cider vinegar
- 1 teaspoon toasted sesame oil
- 1 teaspoon garlic powder
- 1 teaspoon chili powder or smoked or sweet paprika
- ¼ teaspoon freshly ground black pepper
- ¼ teaspoon liquid smoke (optional)
- 1 package (8 ounces) tempeh

1. To make the marinade, put all of the ingredients (except tempeh) in a 8-inch square baking pan and whisk to combine.

2. Cut the block of tempeh into 8 slices lengthwise. Put the tempeh slices into the baking pan and flip over each slice to evenly coat on all sides.

3. Put the baking pan in the refrigerator and let the tempeh marinate for 1 hour or more.

4. Preheat the oven to 400 degrees F. Line a baking sheet with parchment paper or a silicone baking mat.

5. Transfer the tempeh slices to the lined baking sheet. Spoon any remaining marinade over the tempeh slices.

6. Bake for 15 minutes. Remove from the oven. Flip over the tempeh slices with a metal spatula. Bake for 10 to 15 minutes longer, until golden brown and crispy around the edges. Serve hot or cold as desired.

Seitan Sausages

MAKES 4 SERVINGS OR 8 (4-INCH) SAUSAGES

Using vital wheat gluten, rather than whole wheat flour, really speeds up the seitan-making process. With a little effort, you can turn vital wheat gluten and a few seasonings into a tasty batch of vegan sausages that are sure to please. Serve these sausages for breakfast, on sandwiches, or chop or crumble them up for use as a topping or addition to sauces, pizzas, pasta dishes, or casseroles.

- 1¼ cups vital wheat gluten
- ¼ cup chickpea flour
- 2 tablespoons nutritional yeast flakes
- 1½ teaspoons garlic powder
- 1½ teaspoons dried basil
- 1½ teaspoons dried oregano
- 1 teaspoon fennel seeds, or ½ teaspoon ground fennel
- ½ teaspoon crushed red pepper flakes (optional)
- ¼ teaspoon freshly ground black pepper
- 1 cup water or low-sodium vegetable broth
- 1 tablespoon olive oil
- 1 tablespoon reduced-sodium tamari or coconut aminos
- 1 tablespoon maple syrup
- ¼ teaspoon liquid smoke (optional)

1. Set up a large pot with a collapsible steamer basket or steamer rack insert. Add enough water so that it just touches the bottom of the collapsible steamer, or 2 inches deep if using a rack insert. Cover the pot and bring to a boil over medium heat.

2. Put the vital wheat gluten, chickpea flour, nutritional yeast, garlic powder, basil, oregano, fennel seeds, optional red pepper flakes, and pepper in a large bowl and stir to combine.

3. Put the water, oil, tamari, maple syrup, and optional liquid smoke in a medium bowl and stir to combine.

4. Add the water mixture to the vital wheat gluten mixture and stir to combine. Using your hands, knead the mixture in the bowl for 1 to 2 minutes, until the mixture forms a smooth and pliable dough. Let the seitan mixture rest for 5 minutes.

5. Cut 8 (6 x 6-inch) pieces of parchment paper and aluminum foil. Place a piece of parchment paper on top of each piece of aluminum foil, on a work surface, in an assembly line fashion.

6. Place a ¼ cup portion of the sausage mixture lengthwise in the center of each parchment paper. Using your hands, shape each portion into a 4-inch log. Fold over the edges of the parchment paper to enclose the sausage log. Roll up the aluminum foil to enclose the sausage log, and twist the ends to secure (like a piece of wrapped candy).

7. Place the wrapped sausages in the steamer and steam for 25 minutes. Remove from the heat. Let the sausages sit in the steamer for 5 minutes longer. Remove the sausages from the steamer and place them on a large plate. Let the sausages cool for 10 minutes. Remove the sausage wrappers and discard. Serve hot.

Variation: After steaming, the seitan sausages are ready to eat, but, if you prefer, you can cook the sausages further in an oiled skillet (over medium heat) until lightly browned on all sides.

No Eggs Scramble with Chiles and Greens

MAKES 4 SERVINGS

Naturally, eggs are a symbol of fertility, as they often lead to offspring, but there's no need to eat bird eggs. As most veg-heads know, tofu is a great stand-in for eggs when it comes to making a breakfast scramble, and this one is livened up with some jalapeño chiles, onion, and leafy greens.

- 1 pound extra-firm tofu
- 2 tablespoons nutritional yeast flakes
- 1 tablespoon reduced-sodium tamari or coconut aminos
- ½ teaspoon ground turmeric
- ¾ cup diced red or yellow onion
- 2 jalapeño chiles, cut in half lengthwise, seeded, and thinly sliced
- 1 tablespoon olive oil, or ¼ cup low-sodium vegetable broth
- 1 tablespoon minced garlic
- 2 cups kale or mustard greens, stemmed and cut into very thin strips, lightly packed
- ¼ cup chopped fresh basil, cilantro, or parsley, lightly packed
- Sea salt
- Freshly ground black pepper

1. Using your fingers, crumble the tofu into a small bowl. Add the nutritional yeast, tamari, and turmeric and stir to combine.

2. Put the onion, jalapeño chiles, oil (for an oil-free version use vegetable broth), and garlic in a large cast iron or nonstick skillet and cook over medium-high heat, stirring occasionally, for 2 minutes.

3. Add the tofu mixture and cook, stirring occasionally, for 5 minutes.

4. Add the kale and basil and cook, stirring occasionally, for 3 to 5 minutes, until the kale has wilted and the other vegetables are tender. Season with salt and pepper to taste. Serve hot. For extra heat, top servings with a little hot pepper sauce.

Variation: If you're a fan of peppery-tasting arugula, you can replace the kale with 4 cups baby or coarsely chopped arugula, lightly packed.

Herb and Cheese Biscuits

MAKES 6 BISCUITS

Even if you have limited baking experience, you can make these tender biscuits that are enriched with nondairy buttermilk, fragrant fresh herbs, and vegan cheddar cheese. Serve these hard to resist biscuits either plain or topped with vegan butter for breakfast, or as an accompaniment to soups or stews for lunch or dinner.

- ½ cup plain nondairy milk
- 1 tablespoon apple cider vinegar or lemon juice
- 1¾ cups unbleached all-purpose flour or whole wheat pastry flour
- 1 tablespoon aluminum-free baking powder
- 1 tablespoon nutritional yeast flakes
- 1 tablespoon unbleached cane sugar
- ½ teaspoon sea salt
- 3 tablespoons nonhydrogenated vegan butter
- ⅔ cup vegan shredded cheddar cheese
- 2 tablespoons chopped fresh parsley, or 1 tablespoon chopped fresh rosemary

1. Preheat the oven 400 degrees F. Line a baking sheet with parchment paper or a silicone baking mat.

2. Put the milk and vinegar in a small bowl and stir to combine. Let sit for 5 minutes to thicken.

3. Put the flour, baking powder, nutritional yeast flakes, sugar and salt in a medium bowl and stir to combine.

4. Add the vegan butter and use a fork to work it into the flour mixture to form coarse crumbs. Add the milk mixture and stir to combine. Gently stir in the shredded cheese and parsley.

5. Transfer the mixture to the lined baking sheet. Using your hands, gently pat the dough to form a 4 x 6-inch rectangle. Using a sharp knife, cut the rectangle in half widthwise, and then into thirds lengthwise to yield 6 (2-inch) squares. Keep the biscuits shaped as squares, or round the edges with your hands to make them a circular shape as desired.

6. Bake for 8 to 10 minutes, until lightly browned on the bottom and tops are firm to the touch. Serve hot, warm, or at room temperature.

Variation: For a low-fat version, decrease the amount of nondairy milk to ⅓ cup. Replace the vegan butter with ¼ cup plain nondairy yogurt.

Basil and Mozzarella Biscuits: Replace the parsley with 2 tablespoons chopped fresh basil or 2 teaspoons dried basil, and replace the cheddar cheese with ⅔ cup vegan shredded mozzarella cheese.

Sweet Buttermilk Biscuits: Increase the amount of sugar to 2 tablespoons. Omit the chopped parsley and shredded cheese.

Raspberry, Chocolate Chip, and Yogurt Scones

MAKES 8 SCONES

These decadently-rich scones are made with a blend of almond flour, coconut flour, tapioca starch, and nondairy yogurt, and bejeweled with whole raspberries and chocolate chips. Enjoy one of these scones with a cup of tea, coffee, or nondairy milk at any time of the day or night!

- 3 tablespoons warm water
- 1 tablespoon ground gold flaxseeds or gold flaxseed meal
- 2¼ cups blanched almond flour
- ⅓ cup tapioca starch
- 2 tablespoons coconut flour
- 1 teaspoon aluminum-free baking powder
- 1 teaspoon baking soda
- ¼ teaspoon sea salt
- 1 container (6 ounces) plain or vanilla nondairy yogurt
- 1½ tablespoons agave nectar or maple syrup
- 1 teaspoon lemon juice or apple cider vinegar
- 1 teaspoon vanilla extract
- ⅓ cup fresh or frozen raspberries (do not thaw)
- ⅓ cup vegan chocolate chips, or ¼ cup cacao nibs

1. Preheat the oven to 350 degrees F. Line a baking sheet with parchment paper or a silicone baking mat.

2. Put the water and flaxseeds in a small bowl and whisk to combine. Let sit for 10 minutes to thicken into a gel.

3. Put the almond flour, tapioca starch, coconut flour, baking powder, baking soda, and salt in a large bowl and stir to combine.

4. Add the flaxseed mixture, yogurt, agave nectar, lemon juice, and vanilla extract and stir to form a soft dough. Gently stir in the raspberries and chocolate chips.

5. Transfer the dough to the lined baking sheet. Using your hands, gently pat the dough to form a 9-inch circle. Using a sharp knife, cut the circle into 8 wedges, and then gently separate the wedges, spacing them 2 inches apart.

6. Bake for 25 to 30 minutes, until lightly browned around the edges. Let cool for 15 minutes. Serve warm or at room temperature. Store in an airtight container at room temperature or in the refrigerator.

Variation: For a wheat-based version, replace the almond flour, tapioca starch, and coconut flour with 2½ cups unbleached all-purpose flour or whole wheat pastry flour.

Cherry, Chocolate Chip, and Yogurt Scones: Replace the raspberries with ½ cup fresh or frozen (do not thaw) sweet or sour cherries, pitted.

Banana Bread

MAKES 1 (8 X 4 X 2½-INCH) LOAF OR 8 SLICES

When life gives you overripe bananas, why not make banana bread? Using coconut milk or water in the batter is highly recommended, as it heightens the flavor of the loaf. Enjoy slices of this moist, quick bread for breakfast, as a snack, or as a dessert with a scoop of nondairy ice cream and a drizzle of maple syrup.

- 1 large banana, broken into 4 pieces
- ½ cup plain coconut milk beverage or coconut water
- 1 tablespoon sunflower oil or other oil
- 1 tablespoon apple cider vinegar
- 1 teaspoon vanilla extract
- 1½ cups whole wheat pastry flour
- ½ cup unbleached cane sugar or coconut sugar
- 2 teaspoons baking soda
- 1 teaspoon ground cinnamon
- ¼ teaspoon sea salt

1. Preheat the oven to 350 degrees F. Lightly oil a 8 x 4 x 2½-inch loaf pan or mist it with cooking spray.

2. Put the banana in a large bowl and coarsely mash with a fork. Measure out ¾ cup of the mashed banana, and any extra amount can be saved for use in a smoothie (or enjoy as a snack).

3. Add the milk, oil, vinegar, and vanilla extract and whisk to combine.

4. Add the flour, sugar, baking soda, cinnamon, and salt and whisk to combine.

5. Pour the batter into the oiled loaf pan and smooth the top with a spatula.

6. Bake for 25 to 30 minutes, until a toothpick inserted in the center of the loaf comes out clean. Let cool in the pan for 5 minutes. Loosen the sides of the loaf from the pan with a knife. Invert the pan onto a rack and let the loaf release naturally from the pan. Serve warm or at room temperature.

Blueberry-Banana Bread: Add ½ cup fresh or frozen blueberries (do not thaw).

Carrot Cake Muffins
MAKES 6 MUFFINS

All the flavor of a carrot cake, but reimagined in the form of these moist muffins enhanced with grated carrots, chewy raisins and crunchy walnuts. They taste equally delicious served for breakfast, or as a dessert, topped with nondairy yogurt or ice cream.

- 2 tablespoons warm water
- 2 teaspoons ground flaxseeds or flaxseed meal
- 1½ cups blanched almond flour
- 3 tablespoons arrowroot
- 1½ teaspoons aluminum-free baking powder
- 1 teaspoon ground cinnamon
- ½ teaspoon ground ginger
- ¼ teaspoon freshly grated nutmeg
- ¼ teaspoon ground cloves
- ¼ teaspoon sea salt
- 2½ tablespoons plain nondairy milk
- 2½ tablespoons maple syrup
- 1 teaspoon vanilla extract
- ¾ cup coarsely grated carrots, lightly packed
- ¼ cup coarsely chopped raw walnuts
- 2 tablespoon raisins

1. Preheat the oven to 375 degrees F. Line a standard twelve-cup muffin tine with 6 paper or silicone liners, or lightly oil or mist it with cooking spray.

2. Put the water and flaxseeds in a small bowl and whisk to combine. Let sit for 10 minutes to thicken into a gel.

3. Put the almond flour, arrowroot, baking powder, cinnamon, and salt in a large bowl and whisk to combine.

4. Add the flaxseed mixture, milk, maple syrup, and vanilla extract and whisk to combine. Gently stir in the carrots, walnuts, and raisins.

5. Fill the prepared muffin cups using a ¼-cup ice-cream scoop or until three-quarters full. Bake for 22 to 25 minutes, until a toothpick inserted in the center of a muffin comes out clean. Let cool in the pan for 5 minutes, and then transfer to a rack to cool as desired. Serve warm or at room temperature. Store in an airtight container at room temperature or in the refrigerator.

Cappuccino-Chip Muffins

MAKES 6 MUFFINS

Make an extra cup of coffee in the morning and save it to make these moist muffins. Cold coffee and a hint of cacao powder and cinnamon, plus some decadent chocolate chips, come together to create a flavor that's similar to a cappuccino-style beverage.

- 3 tablespoons warm water
- 1 teaspoon chia seeds
- 1 cup unbleached all-purpose flour or whole wheat pastry flour
- 2 tablespoons plus 1½ teaspoons unbleached cane sugar
- 1 tablespoon cacao powder or unsweetened cocoa powder
- 1¼ teaspoons aluminum-free baking powder
- ¼ teaspoon ground cinnamon
- ¼ teaspoon sea salt
- ½ cup cold coffee
- 1½ tablespoons sunflower oil or other oil
- ½ teaspoon vanilla extract
- ½ cup vegan chocolate chips, or ⅓ cup cacao nibs

1. Preheat the oven to 400 degrees F. Line a standard twelve-cup muffin tin with 6 paper or silicone liners, or lightly oil or mist it with cooking spray.

2. Put the water and chia seeds in a small bowl and stir to combine. Let sit for 10 minutes to thicken into a gel.

3. Put the flour, sugar, cacao powder, baking powder, cinnamon, and salt in a medium bowl and whisk to combine.

4. Add the chia seed mixture, coffee, oil, and vanilla extract and whisk to combine. Gently stir in the chocolate chips.

5. Fill the prepared muffin cups using a ¼-cup ice-cream scoop or until three-quarters full. Sprinkle the remaining 1½ teaspoons of sugar over the tops of the muffins. Bake for 18 to 2 minutes, until a toothpick inserted in the center of a muffin comes out clean. Let cool in the pan for 5 minutes, and then transfer to a rack to cool as desired. Serve warm or at room temperature. Store in an airtight container at room temperature or in the refrigerator.

CHAPTER 18

Afternoon Delights-Soups, Salads, and Sandwiches

Married couples with kids often have trouble finding time to fit sex in. Either the kids are always around, or you're driving them to something or other. If you don't have kids in the house, maybe you and your partner have opposite work schedules, and you aren't home at the same time for very long or even at all. Undoubtedly, these are some of the reasons that have lead to the concept of enjoying an afternoon delight with your lover. Of course, after expelling all of that energy during sex, you'll be needing to refuel by having something for lunch. So, whether you're having lunch at home, or taking it with you to-go, these lunch options will fit the bill. Yep, we've got you covered in this chapter with several soups, salads, and sandwiches for satisfying that need.

Gingery Carrot Soup
MAKES 4 SERVINGS

Carrots are an excellent source of beta-carotene, as well as Vitamin C and E. So, if you're feeling a bit under the weather, or in need of a of something that's energizing (yet easy to digest), then make this carrot soup, which is flavored with orange juice, fragrant spices, and lots of fresh ginger.

- 1 pound carrots, sliced
- 4 cups water or low-sodium vegetable broth
- 1 cup diced yellow onion, or 2 medium shallots, diced
- Zest and juice of 1 large orange
- 2 tablespoons peeled and grated fresh ginger
- ¼ teaspoon ground cinnamon
- ¼ teaspoon ground cardamom
- 1½ tablespoons nutritional yeast flakes
- Sea salt

1. Put the carrots, water, onion, orange zest and juice, ginger, cinnamon, and cardamom in a large soup pot and stir to combine. Bring to a boil over high heat. Cover, decrease the heat to low, and simmer for 15 to 20 minutes, until the carrots are tender.

2. Remove from the heat. Let cool for 10 minutes. Transfer half of the soup to a large bowl and set aside. Transfer the other half of the soup to a blender. Add the nutritional yeast and process until smooth. Scrape down the sides of the container with a spatula and process for 15 seconds.

3. Transfer the blended soup back to the soup pot. Place the remaining soup in the blender and process until smooth. Scrape down the sides of the container with a spatula and process for 15 seconds.

4. Transfer the blended soup back to the soup pot. Season with salt to taste. Serve hot.

Variation: For a spicy flavor, replace the cinnamon and cardamom with ½ teaspoon curry powder.

Mexican Tortilla Soup

MAKES 4 SERVINGS

Add a little spice to your day (or night) with a bowl of this colorful, Mexican-style soup! The smoky, tomato-based broth is studded with beans, corn, jalapeño chile, green onions, and cilantro. Then top each serving with crushed tortilla chips, diced avocado, and a squeeze of fresh lime juice.

- 1½ cups low-sodium vegetable broth
- ½ cup diced red onion
- ½ cup thinly sliced green onions
- 1 jalapeño chile, cut in half lengthwise, seeded, and finely diced
- 1 tablespoon minced garlic
- 1 can (28 ounces) crushed tomatoes (preferably fire-roasted)
- 1 can (15 ounces) beans (such as black, pinto, or kidney), drained and rinsed
- ⅔ cup frozen cut corn
- 1½ teaspoons chili powder
- 1 teaspoon ground cumin
- 1 teaspoon dried oregano
- ¼ teaspoon chipotle chile powder or cayenne
- ½ cup chopped fresh cilantro, lightly packed
- Sea salt
- Freshly ground black pepper
- 1 cup coarsely crushed tortilla chips
- 1 avocado, diced
- 1 lime, cut into 4 wedges

1. Put ½ cup of vegetable broth, red onion, green onions, jalapeño chile, and garlic in a large soup pot and cook over medium-high heat, stirring occasionally, for 5 minutes to soften.

2. Add the remaining 1 cup of vegetable broth, crushed tomatoes, beans, corn, chili powder, cumin, oregano, and chipotle chile powder and stir to combine. Bring to a boil over high heat. Cover, decrease the heat to low, and simmer for 15 minutes, until the vegetables are tender.

3. Stir in the cilantro. Season with salt and pepper to taste. Serve hot. Garnish each serving with ¼ cup crushed tortilla chips and one-quarter of the diced avocado, and then squeeze the juice of one lime wedge over the top.

Mood-Enhancing Mushroom Soup

MAKES 4 SERVINGS

Enhance the mood by serving up this soup, which is made by simmering together a combination of aphrodisiacs, including mushrooms, celery, onion, garlic, herbs, and maca powder. Then, to give it a rich and creamy finish, part of the aromatic broth is blended with cashews and white wine.

- 8 ounces (3 cups) mushrooms (such as button, cremini, chanterelle, maitake, or a combination), halved and thinly sliced
- 3 cups low-sodium vegetable broth
- ¾ cup diced celery
- ¾ cup diced yellow onion
- 2 tablespoons minced garlic
- 1 teaspoon dried basil or dried oregano
- 1 teaspoon dried thyme
- ¾ cup raw cashews (soaked for 1 hour or more and drained)
- ¼ cup white wine or dry sherry (optional)
- 2 tablespoons maca powder
- 1½ tablespoons nutritional yeast flakes
- ¼ cup chopped fresh parsley, lightly packed
- Sea salt
- Freshly ground black pepper

1. Put the mushrooms, ½ cup of vegetable broth, celery, onion, garlic, basil, and thyme in a large soup pot and cook over medium-high heat, stirring occasionally, for 5 minutes to soften.

2. Add the remaining 2½ cups of vegetable broth. Bring to a boil over high heat. Cover, decrease the heat to low, and simmer for 20 minutes, until the mushrooms are tender.

3. Transfer 1 cup of the hot soup to a blender. Add the cashews, optional white wine, maca powder, and nutritional yeast and process until smooth.

4. Add the cashew mixture and parsley to the soup pot, stir to combine, and simmer for 2 minutes longer. Season with salt and pepper to taste. Serve hot.

White Bean Chili

MAKES 4 SERVINGS

Not all chilies are red and made with tomatoes. So, if you don't like tomatoes, then give this chili a try, as it's made with white beans, corn, orange bell pepper, and canned green chiles that will get your heart pumping. Serve this hearty chili with tortilla chips, crackers, or cornbread.

- 1 cup diced red or yellow onion
- 1 orange or yellow bell pepper, seeded and diced
- 1 tablespoon olive oil, or ¼ cup water
- 1 tablespoon minced garlic
- 1 teaspoon ground cumin
- 1 teaspoon dried oregano
- ½ teaspoon ground coriander
- 2 cans (15 ounces) white beans (such as Great Northern or navy beans), drained and rinsed
- 3 cups low-sodium vegetable broth
- 1 cup frozen cut corn
- 1 can (4 ounces) green chiles
- ¼ cup chopped fresh cilantro, lightly packed
- 1½ tablespoons nutritional yeast flakes
- Sea salt
- Freshly ground black pepper

1. Put the onions, bell pepper, and oil (for an oil-free version use water) in a large soup pot and cook over medium heat, stirring occasionally, for 5 minutes. Add the garlic, cumin, oregano, and coriander and cook, stirring occasionally, for 1 minute.

2. Put 1 can of white beans and 1 cup of vegetable broth in a food processor and process until smooth.

3. Add the blended mixture, remaining 1 can of white beans, remaining 2 cups of vegetable broth, corn, and green chiles to the soup pot and stir to combine. Cover, decrease the heat to low, and simmer for 20 minutes, until the vegetables are tender.

4. Stir in the cilantro and nutritional yeast. Season with salt and pepper to taste. Serve hot.

Pho You Noodle Bowls

MAKES 4 SERVINGS

This is a veganized version of the popular Vietnamese soup known as Pho, which consists of a savory broth that's enhanced with tofu cubes, leafy greens, chiles, noodles, fresh herbs, and lime juice. The slightly salty, spicy, and citrusy combination of flavors is oh-so-appealing! Plus, you'll have so much fun slurping up the broth-soaked noodles.

- 4 cups low-sodium vegetable broth
- 1 baby bok choy, cut into thin strips, or 2 cups baby spinach, lightly packed
- 1 cup pea pods, cut in half diagonally
- 1 package (6 ounces) smoked or baked tofu, cut into small cubes, or 1 cup firm tofu, cut into small cubes
- 1 jalapeño chile or other chile pepper, cut in half lengthwise and thinly sliced
- 2 tablespoons reduced-sodium tamari or coconut aminos
- 1 tablespoon rice vinegar
- 1 tablespoon peeled and grated fresh ginger
- 1 teaspoon coconut sugar or light brown sugar
- 4 ounces dry rice noodles, buckwheat soba, or other noodles, broken in half
- 1 cup mung bean sprouts
- ¼ cup chopped fresh cilantro or mint, lightly packed
- ¼ cup roasted peanuts, coarsely chopped
- 1 lime, cut into 4 wedges

1. Put vegetable broth, bok choy, pea pods, tofu, jalapeño chile, tamari, vinegar, ginger, and coconut sugar in a large soup pot and stir to combine. Bring to a boil over high heat. Decrease the heat to low and simmer, stirring occasionally, for 5 minutes.

2. Add the noodles and simmer for 2 to 10 minutes (depending on the variety), until the noodles are tender.

3. Stir in the mung bean sprouts and cilantro. Serve hot. Garnish each serving with 1 tablespoon chopped peanuts, and then squeeze the juice of one lime wedge over the top.

Avocado, Fennel, and Citrus Salad
MAKES 2 SERVINGS

For this simple and refreshing salad, thin slices of fennel are briefly marinated in a citrus and mustard vinaigrette to soften its texture and anise-like flavor, then combined with the juicy citrus segments, sliced avocado, and mint leaves.

- 1 large orange or red grapefruit
- 1½ teaspoons olive oil
- ½ teaspoon whole grain mustard or Dijon mustard
- Sea salt
- Freshly ground black pepper
- 1 fennel bulb
- 1 avocado, thinly sliced
- 2 tablespoons mint leaves

1. If using an orange, zest the orange over a large bowl. If using a grapefruit, do not remove the zest. Cut the orange (or grapefruit) into segments, over the bowl with the zest to catch the juices, cut each orange (or grapefruit) segment in half, and set the segments aside.

2. Add the olive oil and mustard to the orange zest and juice and whisk to combine. Season with salt and pepper to taste and set aside.

3. To prepare the fennel, slice off the fronds, coarsely chop them, and set aside. Cut the bulb into quarters lengthwise, remove and discard the core, and then thinly slice each quarter. Add the fennel slices to the orange juice mixture and gently toss to combine. Let the mixture sit for 10 minutes to marinate.

4. Add the reserved chopped fronds and orange (or grapefruit) segments, sliced avocado, and mint leaves and gently toss to combine. Serve immediately.

Variation: For a heartier salad, serve the fennel mixture over 3 cups baby arugula or baby mixed greens, lightly packed.

Greek-Style Chickpea Salad
MAKES 2 SERVINGS

Traditionally, Greek salad is garnished with crumbled pieces of feta cheese, but for this veganized version, this cheesy component is replaced with protein-packed chickpeas. Also, the Greeks believed that eating legumes boosts your libidio. The cooked chickpeas are combined with cubes of cucumber, tomatoes, red onion, olives, and a simple dressing.

- 1 can (15 ounces) chickpeas, drained and rinsed
- 1 cucumber, cut into quarters lengthwise and thickly sliced
- 1 cup halved cherry tomatoes, or 1 cup diced tomatoes
- ½ cup diced red onion
- ⅓ cup pitted Kalamata olives or other black olives, halved
- ¼ cup fresh mint or parsley leaves, lightly packed
- Zest and juice of 1 lemon
- 1 tablespoon olive oil
- 1 tablespoon minced garlic
- 1 teaspoon dried oregano
- Sea salt
- Freshly ground black pepper

1. Put the chickpeas, cucumber, tomatoes, onion, olives, and mint in a large bowl and stir to combine.

2. Add the lemon zest and juice, oil, garlic, and oregano and stir to combine. Season with salt and pepper to taste. Serve immediately.

Fattoush Salad: Lightly toast 1 (6-inch) pita bread, and then tear it into bite-sized pieces. Add the pieces of pita bread to the finished salad and gently stir to combine.

Aphrodite Salad with Pomegranate Dressing

MAKES 2 SERVINGS

Aphrodite, the Greek goddess of beauty and love, is credited with planting the first pomegranate tree, and surely she would approve of this stunning and delicious salad! Tender, baby mixed greens are topped with a combination of fresh berries, dried fruits, and crunchy nuts, and served up with a pink-colored pomegranate dressing.

Pomegranate Dressing:
- ¼ cup pomegranate seeds
- 1½ tablespoons olive oil or walnut oil
- 1 tablespoon apple cider vinegar
- 1 tablespoon agave nectar, maple syrup, or coconut sugar
- 1 tablespoon finely diced shallot or red or yellow onion

Salad:
- 3 cups mixed baby greens, lightly packed
- 1 cup fresh berries (such as blueberries, blackberries, raspberries, or sliced strawberries)
- ½ cup thinly sliced celery
- ¼ cup coarsely chopped dried fruit (such as cherries, cranberries, figs, or pitted soft dates)
- ¼ cup pomegranate seeds
- ¼ cup alfalfa sprouts
- ¼ cup raw sliced almonds or coarsely chopped raw walnuts

1. To make the dressing, put all of the ingredients in a blender and process until smooth. Scrape down the sides of the container with a spatula and process for 15 seconds.

2. To make the salad, put the baby greens, berries, celery, figs, and pomegranate seeds in a large bowl and gently toss to combine. Scatter the alfalfa sprouts and sliced almonds over the top. Serve immediately. Drizzle the pomegranate dressing over individual servings as desired.

Cleopatra Salad with Hemp Seed Dressing

MAKES 2 SERVINGS

Cleopatra is well known for her love affairs with Julius Caesar and Marcus Antony. These tumultuous relationships provided the inspiration for this new take on a tossed Caesar salad, which consists of strips of romaine lettuce, shredded and diced vegetables, and a creamy hemp seed dressing.

Creamy Hemp Seed Dressing:
- 3 tablespoon water
- 2 tablespoons lemon juice
- 1½ tablespoons hemp seeds
- 1 tablespoon raw pine nuts
- ½ teaspoon Dijon mustard
- 1 large clove garlic
- ¼ teaspoon dried basil
- Pinch sea salt
- Pinch freshly ground black pepper

Salad:
- 4 cups romaine lettuce, cut into very thin strips, and lightly packed
- 1½ teaspoons nutritional yeast flakes
- ½ cup shredded beets, lightly packed
- ½ cup shredded carrots, lightly packed
- ½ cup shredded red cabbage, lightly packed
- ½ cup diced zucchini
- ¼ cup toasted pine nuts
- ¼ cup coarsely chopped dried figs

1. To make the dressing, put all of the ingredients in a blender and process until smooth. Scrape down the sides of the container with a spatula and process for 15 seconds.

2. To make the salad, put the lettuce in a large bowl and sprinkle the nutritional yeast over the top. Drizzle the dressing over the mixture and gently toss to combine.

3. Add the beets, carrots, red cabbage, and zucchini and gently toss to combine. Scatter the pine nuts and figs over the top of the salad mixture. Serve immediately.

Pacific Northwest Kale Salad

MAKES 2 SERVINGS

The Pacific Northwest states, Washington and Oregon, are famous for the apples, pears, and hazelnuts (a.k.a. filberts) that are grown there. The crisp and crunchy texture of these highly-prized crops are highlighted in this kale salad, which is cloaked in a piquant apple cider and mustard vinaigrette.

Apple Cider and Mustard Vinaigrette:
- 1 tablespoon apple cider or apple juice
- 1 tablespoon apple cider vinegar
- 2 teaspoons olive oil or hazelnut oil
- 2 teaspoons whole grain mustard, or 1 teaspoon stone ground mustard and ½ teaspoon mustard seeds
- 1 teaspoon chia seeds
- ½ teaspoon agave nectar

Salad:
- 1 medium apple, cored and diced
- 1 medium pear, cored and diced
- 1 teaspoon lemon juice
- 1 bunch green or red-colored kale variety of choice, stemmed and cut into thin strips
- ¼ cup dried cranberries or raisins, or 2 tablespoons dried currants
- ⅓ cup toasted hazelnuts, coarsely chopped

1. To make the dressing, put all of the ingredients in a small bowl and whisk to combine. Let sit for 10 minutes to thicken. Whisk the dressing again to break up any clumps of chia seeds.

2. Put the apple and pear in a small bowl, drizzle the lemon juice over the top, and gently toss to evenly coat.

3. To make the salad, put the kale in a large bowl. Drizzle the dressing over the kale. Using your hands, vigorously massage the kale mixture for 3 to 5 minutes, until the kale begins to wilt.

4. Add the apple-pear mixture, dried cranberries, and hazelnuts, and gently toss to combine. Serve immediately.

Avocado Dream Spread

MAKES 4 SERVINGS

This pale-green spread is made by mashing together avocado and tofu, and then combining it with chopped bits of sun-dried tomatoes, red onion, and bell pepper, along with your choice of vegan yogurt or mayonnaise. Serve generous scoops of this tasty spread on a bed of mixed greens or baby spinach as a salad, or use it as a sandwich filling.

- ⅓ cup hot water
- 5 whole sun-dried tomatoes, or ⅓ cup chopped sun-dried tomato pieces
- 8 ounces firm or extra-firm tofu
- 1 avocado, diced
- 3 tablespoons plain nondairy yogurt or vegan mayonnaise
- 1 tablespoon chopped fresh dill, or 1 teaspoon dried dill weed
- 1 tablespoon nutritional yeast flakes
- 1 tablespoon lemon juice
- 1½ teaspoons reduced-sodium tamari or coconut aminos
- 1 teaspoon garlic powder
- ¼ teaspoon freshly ground black pepper
- ⅓ cup finely diced red onion
- ⅓ cup finely diced orange or red bell pepper

1. Put the water and sun-dried tomatoes in a small bowl. Let sit for 10 minutes to rehydrate and soften the tomatoes. Drain off the soaking liquid. If using whole sun-dried tomatoes, coarsely chop them and set aside.

2. Using your fingers, crumble the tofu into a medium bowl. Add the avocado. Using a potato masher or a fork, mash the tofu and avocado until well combined and slightly smooth.

3. Add the yogurt, dill, nutritional yeast, lemon juice, tamari, garlic powder, and pepper and stir to combine. Add the reserved sun-dried tomatoes, onion, and bell pepper and stir to combine. Serve the spread as a salad topping or sandwich filling as desired. Store in an airtight container in the refrigerator.

Black Bean and Mango Salad Lettuce Wraps

MAKES 4 SERVINGS

Black beans, mango, bell pepper, and red onion come together to create a sweet and slightly spicy salad mixture, which is used to fill large lettuce leaves to create these wrap-style sandwiches. This eye-catching black bean and mango salad is also a great topper for burritos, salads, and cooked grains, or serve it as a dip for tortilla chips.

- 1 can (15 ounces) black beans, drained and rinsed
- 1 mango, peeled, pitted, and diced
- ¾ cup diced red bell pepper
- ½ cup diced red onion
- ¼ cup chopped fresh cilantro, lightly packed
- 1 jalapeño chile, seeded and finely diced
- 1 tablespoon minced garlic
- Juice of 1 lime
- Sea salt
- Freshly ground black pepper
- 4 large Boston or Bibb lettuce leaves or other lettuce leaves

1. To make the salad mixture, put all of the ingredients (except the lettuce leaves) in a medium bowl and stir to combine. Season with salt and pepper to taste.

2. To assemble each lettuce wrap, place a lettuce leaf on a large plate, stem-side up. Spoon ¾ cup of the salad mixture in the center of the leaf. Repeat the process with the remaining lettuce leaves and salad mixture. Serve immediately.

Italian-Style Vegetable Hoagies

MAKES 2 SERVINGS

Hoagie sandwiches (a.k.a. subs) are served up in every neighborhood deli. Usually, these mammoth sandwiches are made with layers of sliced meats, cheeses, and veggies, and they're dripping with an Italian dressing. But not these veg-centric hoagies; they're made by layering vegan cheese slices, an assortment of sliced veggies, and lettuce on split rolls, and then topped as you like with vinegar, olive oil, and seasonings.

- 2 (6-inch) Italian submarine rolls, split, or 4 slices whole grain bread
- 2 large lettuce leaves (such as romaine or green or red-tipped loose-leaf)
- ½ cup thinly sliced orange or red bell pepper
- ¼ cup thinly sliced red or yellow onion
- Olive oil
- Red wine vinegar or balsamic vinegar
- Dried basil and dried oregano
- Sea salt
- Freshly ground black pepper
- Sliced pickles or sliced hot peppers (such as pepperoncini)
- 8 slices tomato
- 4 slices vegan mozzarella cheese or other cheese variety of choice

1. To assemble the hoagies, put the split roll, cut-side-up (or 2 bread slices), on a cutting board. Place one lettuce leaf on the bottom half of each roll (or 1 bread slice). Evenly dividing, put the sliced bell pepper and onion on top of the lettuce.

2. Drizzle a little oil and vinegar over the vegetables as desired. Season with dried basil, dried oregano, salt, and pepper to taste.

3. Top with sliced pickles (or hot peppers) as desired. Evenly dividing, layer the tomato and cheese slices on top. Replace the top half of the roll (or top with remaining slice of bread), and then carefully cut in half if desired. Serve immediately, or to take-them-to-go, wrap them with plastic wrap or place them in an airtight container and store in the refrigerator.

Chocolate-Nut Butter Spread and Banana Paninis

MAKES 2 SANDWICHES

Pairing chocolate and banana together is a combination that appeals to both kids and adults alike. No matter what your age, you're sure to love these hot, panini-style sandwiches, which can be served up for any meal of the day or as a snack.

Chocolate-Nut Butter Spread:
- ¼ cup nut butter (such as almond, cashew, or peanut)
- 1½ tablespoons cacao powder or unsweetened cocoa powder
- 1 tablespoon maple syrup or agave nectar

- ½ teaspoon vanilla extract
- 4 slices whole grain bread
- 1 medium banana, thinly sliced
- 4 teaspoons softened nonhydrogenated vegan butter or melted coconut oil

---

1. To make the chocolate-nut butter spread, put the nut butter, cacao powder, maple syrup, and vanilla extract in a small bowl and stir to combine.

2. To assemble the paninis, place the bread slices on a cutting board. Spread 1 tablespoon of the chocolate-nut butter spread on each slice of bread. Evenly layer half of the sliced banana on top of two of the spread-covered slices of bread, and then top with the remaining two spread-covered slices of bread, spread-side-in.

3. Preheat a panini maker to medium-high heat. Alternatively, use a large cast iron or nonstick skillet and place over to medium-high heat.

4. To cook the paninis, spread 1 teaspoon of vegan butter on the top of each assembled sandwich. Place margarine-side-down in the panini maker (or skillet), and spread another 1 teaspoon of vegan butter on the top of each sandwich. Close the panini maker and cook for 3 to 5 minutes, until the bread is golden brown. Alternatively, if using

a skillet, cook for 3 minutes per side. Cut each sandwich in half if
desired. Serve hot.

Variation: Replace the sliced banana on each sandwich with ⅓ cup raspberries
or sliced strawberries.

Baked Falafel and Cucumber Tzatziki Pita Sandwiches

MAKES 4 SERVINGS

Chickpea-based falafel is so addictively delicious! That being said, eating too many fried falafel can leave you feeling heavy and sluggish, but you won't have that problem if you make these oven-baked and oil-free ones instead. Use whole pita bread to hold the cooked falafel balls and veggie fixings, and then top them with the creamy yogurt-based, cucumber tzatziki sauce.

Baked Falafel:
- ½ a small yellow onion
- 4 large cloves garlic
- ¼ cup fresh parsley or cilantro leaves (or a combination), lightly packed
- Zest and juice of ½ a lemon
- 1 teaspoon ground cumin
- 1 teaspoon ground coriander
- ½ teaspoon sea salt
- ¼ teaspoon freshly ground black pepper
- 1 can (15 ounces) chickpeas, drained and rinsed
- ¼ cup chickpea flour or whole wheat flour
- 1 teaspoon baking powder

Cucumber Tzatziki:
- 1 container (6 ounces) plain nondairy yogurt
- ¼ cup finely diced cucumber
- 1 tablespoon chopped fresh mint or dill
- Sea salt
- Freshly ground black pepper
- 4 pita breads
- 4 large lettuce leaves (such as romaine or green or red-tipped loose-leaf)
- 1 large tomato, diced

1. Preheat the oven to 400 degrees F. Line a baking sheet with parchment paper or a silicone baking mat.

2. To make the baked falafel, put the onion, garlic, parsley, lemon zest and juice, cumin, coriander, salt, and pepper in a food processor and process until finely chopped. Scrape down the sides of the container with a spatula. Add the chickpeas, flour, and baking powder and process until the mixture is coarsely chopped (do not purée). Cover and refrigerate for 30 minutes to let the falafel mixture firm up slightly.

3. Using a 1½-inch ice-cream scoop or a heaping tablespoonful for each, portion the falafel mixture, spacing them 2 inches apart, and it should make 12 portions. Leave the falafel ball-shaped or slightly flatten each ball with your fingers.

4. Bake the falafel for 15 minutes. Remove from the oven. Flip the falafel over with a metal spatula. Bake the falafel for 10 to 12 minutes longer, until golden brown on both sides.

5. While the falafels are baking, make the cucumber tzatziki. Put all of the ingredients in a small bowl and stir to combine. Season with salt and pepper to taste.

6. To assemble each pita sandwich, place a pita bread on a large plate, bottom-side-up. Place one lettuce leaf horizontally in the center of the pita bread. Place 3 falafels on top of the lettuce. Then top with one-quarter of the cucumber tzatziki and one-quarter of the diced tomatoes. Repeat the assembly procedure with the remaining ingredients.

7. Fold the assembled pita sandwiches like a taco to eat. Serve immediately, or to take-them-to-go, wrap them with plastic wrap or place them in an airtight container and store in the refrigerator.

Quarter Pounder Beet Burgers

MAKES 4 BURGERS

These crimson-colored burgers are made with a savory blend of seasonings, beets, and your choice of quinoa or millet, plus some coarsely ground walnuts for a little added texture and protein. Also, the boron and tryptophan in the beets will increases your body's sex hormones and make feel more relaxed and aroused at the same time. Serve them on plates, burger buns, or sliced bread with your favorite condiments and toppings.

- 1¼ cups water
- 1 cup shredded beets, lightly packed
- ½ cup quinoa or millet, rinsed
- ½ cup finely diced red or yellow onion
- 4 large cloves garlic, minced
- 1½ teaspoons Italian seasonings blend, or ½ teaspoon each dried basil, oregano, and rosemary
- ¾ teaspoon ground cumin
- ½ teaspoon chili powder, or ½ teaspoon smoked or sweet paprika
- 1½ tablespoons ground flaxseeds or flaxseed meal
- ½ cup coarsely ground raw walnuts
- 1½ tablespoons nutritional yeast flakes
- Sea salt
- Freshly ground black pepper

1. Put 1 cup water, beets, quinoa, onion, garlic, Italian seasonings blend, cumin, and chili powder in a large saucepan and stir to combine. Bring to a boil over high heat. Cover, decrease the heat to low, and simmer for 20 to 25 minutes, until the quinoa is tender and all of the water is absorbed. Remove from the heat and uncover the saucepan. Let cool for 10 minutes.

2. Put the remaining ¼ cup water and flaxseeds in a small bowl and stir to combine. Let sit for 10 minutes to thicken into a gel.

3. Transfer the beet mixture to a large bowl. Add the flaxseed mixture, walnuts, and nutritional yeast. Using a spoon or fork, stir to combine and slightly mash the burger mixture against the side of the bowl to bind it together. Season with salt and pepper to taste.

4. Line a baking sheet with parchment paper or a silicone baking mat. Using a ½ cup measuring cup, portion each patty by lightly filling and gently packing the burger mixture into the cup with the back of a spoon. Flip the measuring cup over onto the lined baking sheet and tap the cup to release the burger mixture. Slightly flatten each portion into a patty. Refrigerate the patties for at least 1 hour to let them firm up slightly.

5. Preheat the oven to 400 degrees F. Bake the burgers for 15 minutes. Remove from the oven. Flip the burgers over with a metal spatula. Bake the burgers for 15 to 20 minutes longer, until golden brown on both sides. Serve the burgers plain on plates, or on burger buns or sliced bread with your choice of condiments and toppings. Serve immediately, or to take-them-to-go, wrap them with plastic wrap or place them in an airtight container and store in the refrigerator.

Beet Sliders: Use a ¼ cup measuring cup to portion each patty. Bake for 10 minutes, flip the burgers over, and bake for 10 to 12 minutes longer, until golden brown on both sides.

CHAPTER 19

Naughty Nibbles–Snacks and Appetizers

Eating between meals has become the norm for most of us in our day-to-day lives. Many nutrition experts say that it's better for your metabolism to eat several times throughout the day, rather than just eating three big meals. Maybe you need a little snack after sex? Or perhaps, something to whet (no, it's not *wet*) your appetite? We all have those times when we're craving something to nibble on, you know, to tide you over for awhile. So look to this chapter when you're in need of a sweet or savory snack, tasty spread or dunkable dip, bite-sized morsel, or an appealing appetizer.

Bliss Balls

MAKES 4 SERVINGS OR 12 BALLS

Are you in need of an energizing snack that's good for you? Just make a batch of these naturally-sweetened bliss balls. They're made with a combination of dried fruit, walnuts, and shredded coconut, a little bit of coconut water, chia seeds, and maca powder (if you like), and then the shaped balls are coated in additional shredded coconut.

- 3 tablespoons coconut water or water
- 1 teaspoon chia seeds
- ¾ cup raw walnuts
- ½ cup raisins
- ½ cup pitted soft dates
- ½ cup dried fruit (such as cherries, cranberries, currants, chopped dates, chopped figs, chopped apricots, or a combination)
- ½ cup unsweetened shredded dried coconut, plus additional for coating
- 1½ tablespoons maca powder (optional)
- 1 teaspoon vanilla extract

1. Put the coconut water and chia seeds in a small bowl and stir to combine. Let sit for 10 minutes to thicken into a gel.

2. Put the walnuts in a food processor and process until finely chopped. Transfer to a small plate.

3. Put the raisins, dates, and dried fruit in the food processor and process for 1 to 2 minutes, until finely chopped. Add the chia seed mixture, reserved walnuts, coconut, optional maca powder, and vanilla extract, and process for 1 to 2 minutes, until the mixture comes together to form a ball.

4. Place some additional shredded coconut on a small plate. Dampen your hands with water, roll the fruit mixture into 12 (1-inch) balls, and then roll each ball in shredded coconut until evenly coated on all sides. Store in an airtight container in the refrigerator or freezer.

Apricot Delights

MAKES 4 SERVINGS OR 12 BALLS

Turkish Delight is a candy-like confection that is traditionally made with a gelled mixture of chopped dates and pistachios (or other nuts) and then coated with a powdery starch. Taking inspiration from these candies, these finger-sized treats are made with a blend of dried fruits, nuts, seeds, and a mandarin or satsuma orange.

- 1 medium mandarin or satsuma orange
- 3 tablespoons raw whole almonds
- 1½ tablespoons unsweetened shredded dried coconut
- ½ cup raw pistachios
- 2 tablespoons hemp seeds
- ¾ cup dried apricots
- ½ cup pitted soft dates
- ¾ teaspoon ground cinnamon

1. Zest the orange and set aside. Juice the orange, measure out 4 teaspoons of juice, and set aside.

2. Put the almonds in a food processor and process until coarsely chopped. Scrape down the sides of the container with a spatula. Add the reserved orange zest and coconut and process for 1 minute, until the mixture is finely chopped. Transfer the almond mixture to a small plate and set aside.

3. Put the pistachios in the food processor and process until coarsely chopped. Transfer to a medium bowl. Stir in the hemp seeds.

4. Put the apricots, dates, reserved orange juice, and cinnamon in the food processor and process for 1 to 2 minutes, until the mixture comes together to form a ball.

5. Add the apricot mixture to the pistachio mixture. Using your hands, knead the two mixtures together until well combined. Flatten the mixture in the bowl. Using a sharp knife, cut the mixture into 12 wedges.

6. To assemble the apricot delights, dampen your hands with water, roll each wedge into a 1 x 2-inch log, and place them on a large plate. Roll each log in the reserved almond-coconut mixture until evenly coated on all sides. Store in an airtight container in the refrigerator or freezer.

Cinnamon and Vanilla-Kissed Almonds

MAKES 6 (¼ CUP) SERVINGS

Some people have a placard or apron in their kitchen that says, "Kiss the Cook!," and you're sure to get a few kisses from your lover after they sample these sweetened and spiced almonds.

- 1½ cups raw whole almonds
- 1 tablespoon vanilla extract
- 1½ teaspoons powdered sugar
- 1½ teaspoons ground cinnamon

1. Preheat the oven to 375 degrees F. Line a baking sheet with parchment paper or a silicone baking mat.

2. Place the almonds on the lined baking sheet. Bake for 5 to 7 minutes, until the almonds are lightly toasted and fragrant.

3. Immediately, transfer the toasted almonds to a medium bowl. Add the vanilla extract (it will make a sizzling sound) and stir to evenly coat the almonds.

4. Put the powdered sugar and cinnamon in a small bowl and stir to combine. Sprinkle the cinnamon-sugar mixture over the almonds and gently toss to evenly coat the almonds with the mixture. Store in an airtight container at room temperature.

Chai-Kissed Almonds: Decrease the amount of cinnamon to ¾ teaspoon, and add ½ teaspoon ground cardamom and ¼ teaspoon ground ginger.

Variation: Feel free to replace the almonds with other toasted nuts (such as cashews, walnuts, or pecans).

Cocoa-Coated Cashews

MAKES 6 (¼ CUP) SERVINGS

Toasted cashews are double coated with melted chocolate chips and then dusted with cocoa powder to create these delectable morsels. Enjoy them by the handful, or use them as a topping for nondairy ice cream.

- 1½ cups raw cashews
- ¾ cup vegan chocolate chips
- 1 tablespoon plain or vanilla nondairy milk
- ½ teaspoon vanilla extract
- 1 ½ tablespoons cacao powder or unsweetened cocoa powder

1. Preheat the oven to 375 degrees F. Line a baking sheet with parchment paper or a silicone baking mat.

2. Place the cashews on the lined baking sheet. Bake for 5 to 7 minutes, until the cashews are golden brown and fragrant. Let cool completely.

3. Put the chocolate chips, milk, and vanilla extract in a medium bowl and put in the microwave for 1 to 2 minutes to melt the chips. Alternatively, put the chocolate chip mixture in a double boiler over medium-low heat until the chips are melted.

4. Add the toasted cashews to the melted chocolate chip mixture and stir to evenly coat the cashews.

5. Using a slotted spoon or fork, remove the cashews from the chocolate chip mixture, and place them individually back onto the lined baking sheet. Reserve the melted chocolate chip mixture.

6. Refrigerate the cashews for 15 minutes. Repeat the chocolate coating and refrigerating procedures.

7. Put the cacao powder in a medium bowl. Add the cashews and gently toss to evenly coat the cashews with cocoa powder. Store in an airtight container in the refrigerator.

Variation: Feel free to replace the cashews with other toasted nuts (such as almonds, hazelnuts, or pecans).

Sweet and Savory Snack Mix

MAKES 8 (¼ CUP) SERVINGS

Sometimes you're not quite sure what you're in the mood to snack on, and you find yourself going back and forth as to whether it's something sweet or savory that you desire. Perhaps it's both of these tastes that you're longing for, and if that's the case, then this quick snack mix is just the thing you need to satisfy your cravings for something sweet and savory to nibble on.

- 1 recipe Coconut Bacon (see Avocado Toast with Coconut Bacon in Morning Quickies)
- ½ cup banana chips
- ½ cup roasted peanuts
- ½ cup vegan chocolate chips

1. Prepare the coconut bacon according to the recipe instructions. Let cool completely.

2. Transfer the cooled coconut bacon to a medium bowl. Add the remaining ingredients and stir to combine. Store in an airtight container at room temperature.

Santa Fe Trail Mix
MAKES 8 (¼ CUP) SERVINGS

Those who love crunchy snacks, and the smoky flavors of Southwest cuisine, will find the taste of this trail mix quite addictive! This colorful, hand-to-mouth trail mix is made with well-seasoned mixed nuts, seeds, and pretzels, which, after baking, are combined with fiery-red goji berries and chewy pieces of dried mango and dates.

- ½ teaspoon chili powder or chipotle chile powder
- ½ teaspoon garlic powder
- ½ teaspoon ground coriander
- ½ teaspoon ground cumin
- ½ teaspoon dried oregano
- ½ teaspoon smoked or sweet paprika
- 1 tablespoon lime juice
- 1½ teaspoons olive oil
- 1½ teaspoons reduced-sodium tamari or coconut aminos
- ½ cup pretzels (preferably nuggets or tiny twists variety)
- ⅓ cup raw whole almonds
- ⅓ cup raw pecans
- ⅓ cup raw pumpkin seeds
- ¼ cup raw pine nuts
- ⅓ cup coarsely chopped dried mango
- ⅓ cup date pieces covered with oat flour
- ⅓ cup goji berries

1. Preheat the oven to 350 degrees F. Line a baking sheet with parchment paper or a silicone baking mat.

2. Put the chili powder, garlic powder, coriander, cumin, oregano, and paprika in a small bowl and stir to combine.

3. Put the lime juice, oil, and tamari in a medium bowl and stir to combine.

4. Add the pretzels, almonds, pecans, pumpkin seeds, and pine nuts and stir to combine. Sprinkle the reserved spice mixture over the top and stir to evenly coat the pretzel mixture.

5. Transfer the pretzel mixture to lined baking sheet and spread into a single layer. Bake for 10 to 15 minutes, until the mixture is lightly toasted and fragrant. Let cool completely.

6.   Transfer the cooled pretzel mixture to a medium bowl. Add the remaining ingredients and stir to combine. Store in an airtight container at room temperature.

Lemon-Herb Roasted Chickpeas

MAKES 4 (⅓ CUP) SERVINGS

Roasted chickpeas are all the rage, and understandably so, as they're one tasty, protein-packed snack! It's truly hard to believe that seasoning cooked chickpeas and baking them off magically transforms them into crunchy munchables.

- 1 can (15 ounces) chickpeas, drained and rinsed
- 1 tablespoon lemon juice
- 2 teaspoons agave nectar or maple syrup
- 2 teaspoons olive oil (optional)
- 1½ teaspoons nutritional yeast flakes
- 1½ teaspoons Italian seasonings blend, or ½ teaspoon each dried basil, oregano, and rosemary
- 1½ teaspoons garlic powder
- ½ teaspoon smoked or sweet paprika

1. Put the chickpeas on a clean kitchen towel or paper towels, and allow to air dry for 10 minutes.

2. Preheat the oven to 425 degrees F. Line a baking sheet with parchment paper or a silicone baking mat.

3. Put the lemon juice, agave nectar, oil, nutritional yeast, Italian seasonings blend, garlic powder, and paprika in a small bowl and stir to combine. Add the chickpeas and stir to evenly coat the chickpeas with the lemon juice mixture.

4. Transfer the chickpea mixture to the lined baking sheet and spread them into a single layer. Bake for 25 to 30 minutes, shaking the pan every 10 minutes to ensure even baking, until the chickpeas are golden brown, dry, and slightly crunchy.

Chile-Lime Roasted Chickpeas: Replace the lemon juice with 1 tablespoon lime juice. Replace the olive oil with 1 teaspoon reduced-sodium tamari or coconut aminos and 1 teaspoon toasted sesame oil. Replace the Italian seasonings blend with ½ teaspoon chili powder, ½ teaspoon ground cumin, and ¼ teaspoon chipotle chile powder or cayenne.

Fruit-n-Nut Crackers

MAKES 48 (1½-INCH) CRACKERS

Both almond flour and almond meal are combined with chopped sunflower seeds and dried currants to create these sweet and nutty flavored crackers. Serve them plain or topped with slices of vegan cheese, and they pair quite nicely with a glass of wine.

- 1 cup almond flour
- 1 cup almond meal
- 1 tablespoon dried basil or dried thyme
- ¾ teaspoon sea salt
- ¼ cup water
- 1½ tablespoons sunflower oil or other oil
- ¼ cup coarsely chopped raw sunflower seeds
- 2 tablespoons dried currants

1. Preheat the oven to 300 degrees F. Line a baking sheet with parchment paper or a silicone baking mat.

2. Put the almond flour, almond meal, basil, and salt in a medium bowl and stir to combine.

3. Add the water and oil and stir to combine. Add the sunflower seeds and currants and stir until the mixture comes together to form a soft dough.

4. Transfer the dough to the lined baking sheet. Place another sheet of parchment paper (or silicone baking mat) on top. Using a rolling pin, roll the dough into a 9 x 12-inch rectangle, about ⅛-inch thick.

5. Remove the top sheet of parchment paper. Using a sharp knife or pizza cutter, cut the dough into 1½-inch squares.

6. Bake for 18 to 22 minutes, until the crackers feel dry and are lightly browned around the edges. Watch closely during the last 2 minutes of baking time to avoid burning them. Let cool completely on the baking sheet. Store in an airtight container at room temperature or in the refrigerator.

Variation: Replace the dried currants with 2 tablespoons finely chopped dried cranberries, raisins, or pitted soft dates.

Super Seed Crackers: Omit the dried basil and currants. Decrease the amount of chopped sunflower seeds to 2 tablespoons, and then add 2 tablespoons each of hemp seeds, sesame seeds, and coarsely chopped raw pumpkin seeds.

Artichoke Pâté

MAKES 4 SERVINGS

Artichokes are often paired with lemons, as their flavors not only complement each other, but lemon juice also helps to prevent them from turning brown. For this Romanesque recipe, almonds, pine nuts, artichokes, and lemon zest and juice are blended to create a palatable pâté, which can be served as a spread or dip for raw or cooked veggies, crackers, bread slices, or sandwiches.

- ½ cup raw whole almonds (soaked for 1 hour or more and drained)
- 2 tablespoons raw pine nuts
- ¾ cup canned or frozen artichoke hearts (thawed), each heart quartered
- 2 tablespoons water
- Zest and juice of ½ a lemon
- 1 tablespoon nutritional yeast flakes
- 1 tablespoon minced garlic
- Sea salt

1. Squeeze each almond between your thumb and forefinger to remove the skin. Put the almonds and pine nuts in a food processor and process until finely ground. Scrape down the sides of the container with a spatula.

2. Add the remaining ingredients and process until smooth. Season with salt to taste and process for 15 seconds longer. Store in an airtight container in the refrigerator.

Kalamata Olive Hummus
MAKES 6 (¼ CUP) SERVINGS

Slight salty Kalamata olives and tangy, aged balsamic vinegar come together to create a wonderful contrast of flavors in this sophisticated version of a traditional hummus. Serve this versatile dip with pita bread, crackers, or raw vegetables, or use as a filling for wraps and sandwiches.

- ½ cup Kalamata olives or other olives variety of choice, pitted
- 1 can (15 ounces) chickpeas, drained and rinsed
- 4 large cloves garlic
- 2 tablespoons balsamic vinegar
- 2 tablespoons lemon juice
- 2 tablespoons tahini
- ½ teaspoon ground cumin
- Sea salt
- Freshly ground black pepper
- Sweet or smoked paprika (optional)

1. Put the olives in a food processor and pulse until coarsely chopped. Put half of the chopped olives in a small bowl and set aside.

2. Add the chickpeas and garlic to the food processor and process for 1 minute.

3. Add the vinegar, lemon juice, tahini, and cumin and process until smooth. Scrape down the sides of the container with a spatula. Season with salt and pepper to taste and process for 15 seconds longer.

4. Transfer the hummus to an airtight container. Stir in the reserved chopped olives. Sprinkle a little paprika over the top if desired. Store in an airtight container in the refrigerator.

Whoo-Pea Guacamole with Baked Tortilla Chips

MAKES 4 SERVINGS (⅓ CUP GUACAMOLE AND 6 CHIPS)

You can significantly cut the fat content of guacamole by blending the avocado with some peas, and doing so will also add a bit of sweetness and keep the color a vibrant green as well. Also included are instructions for transforming corn tortillas into a batch of homemade tortilla chips, which bake up light and crispy without adding oil. If you're feeling a little lazy, you can enjoy the guacamole with store-bought tortilla chips.

- 4 (6-inch) corn tortillas
- 1 avocado, cut in half
- 1 cup frozen peas (thawed)
- 2 large cloves garlic, minced
- 1½ teaspoons nutritional yeast flakes
- ½ teaspoon chili powder, or ¼ teaspoon hot pepper sauce
- Juice of ½ a lime
- 1 jalapeño chile or serrano chile, seeded and finely diced
- ¼ cup finely diced tomatoes
- 2 tablespoons finely diced red or yellow onion
- 2 tablespoons chopped fresh cilantro
- Sea salt
- Freshly ground black pepper

1. To make the baked tortilla chips, preheat the oven to 350 degrees F. Line a baking sheet with parchment paper or a silicone baking mat.

2. Stack the tortillas on top of each other, and then cut them into 6 wedges. Arrange the cut wedges in a single layer on the lined baking sheet.

3. Bake for 8 to 10 minutes, until the chips are crisp. Watch closely during the last 2 minutes of baking time to avoid burning them.

4. To make the guacamole, put the avocado, peas, jalapeño chile, garlic, nutritional yeast, chili powder, and lime juice in a food processor and process until smooth. Scrape down the sides of the container with a spatula and process for 15 seconds longer.

5. Transfer the avocado mixture to a small bowl. Add the tomatoes, onion, and cilantro and stir to combine. Season with salt and pepper to taste. Serve the guacamole with the warm or room temperature tortilla chips. Store the tortilla chips in an airtight container at room temperature, and store the guacamole in an airtight container in the refrigerator.

Papaya-Pineapple Salsa

MAKES 6 (⅓ CUP) SERVINGS

Juicy pieces of papaya and pineapple are the stars in this sweet and slightly spicy salsa, which can be used as a dipper for store-bought tortilla chips or the Baked Tortilla Chips (see Whoo-Pea Guacamole with Baked Tortilla Chips recipe in this chapter). This tropical-tasting salsa is also a great topper for burritos, salads, and cooked black beans.

- 1 medium papaya, peeled, seeded, and diced
- ½ cup canned or frozen (thawed) pineapple tidbits
- ¾ cup diced red bell pepper
- ½ cup diced red onion
- ¼ cup chopped fresh cilantro, lightly packed
- 1 jalapeño chile, seeded and finely diced
- 1 tablespoon minced garlic
- Juice of 1 lime
- Sea salt
- Freshly ground black pepper

1. Put all of the ingredients in a medium bowl and stir to combine. Season with salt and pepper to taste. Serve immediately. Store in an airtight container in the refrigerator.

Mango-Pineapple Salsa: Replace the papaya with 2 mangoes, peeled, pitted, and diced.

Smoked Cheddar Cashew Cheese Ball

MAKES 4 SERVINGS

For some, a party isn't a party unless there's a nut-crusted cheese ball. And yes, it can be just a two-person party if you want. Just because you've gone dairy-free, it doesn't mean that you have to go without, as this smoked cheddar-tasting cheese ball is made with soaked cashews and a few other ingredients. Serve the cheese ball with crackers or toasted bread slices.

- 1 cup raw cashews (soaked in water for 1 hour or more and drained)
- ½ of a red bell pepper, seeded and diced
- ¼ cup nutritional yeast flakes
- 2 tablespoon lemon juice
- 1 teaspoon Dijon mustard
- ½ teaspoon garlic powder
- ½ teaspoon onion powder
- ½ teaspoon smoked or sweet paprika
- ½ teaspoon sea salt
- ⅛ teaspoon chipotle chile powder, cayenne, or hot pepper sauce
- ⅓ cup toasted pecans or walnuts, coarsely chopped

1. Put the cashews, bell pepper, nutritional yeast, lemon juice, mustard, garlic powder, onion powder, paprika, salt, and chipotle chile powder in a food processor and process until smooth. Scrape down the sides of the container with a spatula and process for 15 seconds longer.

2. Place the cashew mixture in the center of a piece of plastic wrap (at least 8 inches in length). Gently wrap the plastic wrap around the mixture, and then use your hands to shape it into a ball. Refrigerate the covered cheese ball for 4 hours or more.

3. Remove the plastic wrap and place the cheese ball on a plate. Press the toasted pecans into the cheese ball to evenly coat on all sides. Cover the cheese ball with clean plastic wrap and refrigerate until ready to serve. Serve cold or at room temperature as desired.

Variation: For a mild cheddar taste, use sweet paprika and omit the chipotle chile powder.

Hot Artichoke and Spinach Dip

MAKES 6 SERVINGS

The classic spinach and artichoke dip gets a vegan makeover. This creamy dip is made with a savory mix of spinach, artichoke hearts, onion, and garlic, along with a lemon-accented vegan mozzarella cheese sauce. Serve it with thin slices of bread, crackers, or vegetable crudités.

- ⅓ cup finely diced yellow onion
- 1 teaspoon olive oil
- 2 cups finely chopped baby spinach, lightly packed
- 1½ tablespoons minced garlic
- 1 can (14 ounces) artichoke hearts packed in water, drained and coarsely chopped
- 1⅓ cups plain nondairy milk
- 3 tablespoons nutritional yeast flakes
- 2 tablespoons tapioca starch
- Zest and juice of 1 lemon
- 1 teaspoon Dijon mustard
- 1 teaspoon dried basil
- ½ teaspoon sea salt
- ½ teaspoon crushed red pepper flakes
- ¼ teaspoon freshly ground black pepper
- ⅔ cup vegan shredded mozzarella cheese
- Smoked or sweet paprika

1. Preheat the oven to 400 degrees F. Lightly oil a 8-inch baking pan or mist it with cooking spray.

2. Put the onion and oil in a large cast iron or nonstick skillet and cook over medium-high heat, stirring occasionally, for 3 minutes.

3. Add the spinach and garlic and cook, stirring occasionally, for 2 to 3 minutes, until the spinach is tender. Stir in the artichoke hearts. Transfer the spinach mixture to the oiled baking pan.

4. Put the milk, nutritional yeast, tapioca starch, lemon zest and juice, mustard, basil, salt, red pepper flakes, and pepper in a blender and process until smooth. Scrape down the sides of the container with a spatula and process for 15 seconds longer.

5. Add the milk mixture and shredded cheese to the baking pan and stir to combine. Sprinkle a little paprika over the top as desired.

6. Bake for 25 to 30 minutes, until the dip is hot and bubbly around the edges. Serve hot with thin slices of bread, crackers, or vegetable crudités.

Cucumber Canapés with Red Pepper Spread

MAKES 4 SERVINGS

Canapés are finger-foods that are usually made on small slices of bread or crackers. For this lighter version, thick slices of cucumber are utilized as the sturdy base for a creamy red pepper spread.

- ⅔ cup diced red bell pepper
- 2 large cloves garlic
- 1 tablespoon lemon juice
- 1 tablespoon water
- ½ cup raw cashews or raw pine nuts (soaked for 1 hour or more and drained)
- 2 tablespoons nutritional yeast flakes
- ½ teaspoon smoked or sweet paprika
- ⅛ teaspoon cayenne or hot pepper sauce
- Sea salt
- 1 large cucumber, cut into 16 thick slices
- Fresh parsley or dill sprigs

1. To make the red pepper spread, put the bell pepper, garlic, lemon juice, and water in a food processor and process for 1 minute, until finely chopped. Scrape down the sides of the container with a spatula.

2. Add the cashews, nutritional yeast, paprika, and cayenne and process until smooth. Season with salt to taste and process for 15 seconds longer.

3. To make the canapés, place the cucumber slices on a large plate or platter. Top each cucumber slice with 1 tablespoon of the red pepper spread. Garnish each canapé with a small sprig of parsley or dill as desired. Serve immediately.

Cucumber Canapés with Sun-Dried Tomato Spread: Omit the red bell pepper. When soaking the cashews, also add 3 whole sun-dried tomatoes.

Crispy Buffalo Cauliflower with Ranch Dressing

MAKES 4 SERVINGS

Cauliflower florets are first cloaked in a hot pepper sauce-spiked batter, then coated with a generously-spiced breading, and baked until golden brown and crispy. To offset the fiery flavor of these cauliflower morsels, they're served with a thick and creamy, dairy-free ranch dressing.

Ranch Dressing:
- ¾ cup plain soy milk or other nondairy milk
- 2 tablespoons chopped fresh parsley
- 1 tablespoon apple cider vinegar
- 1 tablespoon nutritional yeast flakes
- 1½ teaspoons chia seeds
- ½ teaspoon dried dill weed
- ½ teaspoon dried thyme
- ½ teaspoon garlic powder
- ½ teaspoon onion powder

Batter:
- ½ cup plain soy milk or other nondairy milk
- ¼ cup blanched almond flour
- ¼ cup cornstarch
- 2 tablespoons hot pepper sauce

- 1½ teaspoons apple cider vinegar
- 1½ teaspoons chili powder
- ½ teaspoon garlic powder
- ½ teaspoon sea salt
- ½ teaspoon freshly ground black pepper
- 4 cups (1 medium) cauliflower, cut into small florets

Breading:
- ½ cup almond flour
- ⅓ cup chickpea flour
- 2 tablespoons cornstarch
- 1 tablespoons nutritional yeast flakes
- 1½ teaspoons chili powder
- 1 teaspoon garlic powder
- 1 teaspoon onion powder
- 1 teaspoon chipotle chile powder or cayenne
- ½ teaspoon sea salt

1. To make the ranch dressing, put all of the ingredients in a blender and process until smooth. Scrape down the sides of the container with a spatula and let sit for 10 minutes. Process again for 15 seconds to break up any clumps of chia seeds. Transfer the mixture to an airtight container and refrigerate for 30 minutes to thicken the ranch dressing.

2.   To make the batter, put all of the ingredients (except the cauliflower) in a large bowl and whisk to form a thick batter. Add the cauliflower, stir until evenly coated, and allow the cauliflower to marinate for 15 minutes, stirring every 5 minutes.

3.   Preheat the oven to 450 degrees F. Line a baking sheet with parchment paper or a silicone baking mat.

4.   To make the breading, put all of the ingredients in a large zipper-lock bag (or container with a tight fitting lid) and shake until well combined. Add the cauliflower to the bag and shake until evenly coated.

5.   Place the cauliflower in a single layer on the lined baking sheet. Lightly drizzle a little olive oil over the cauliflower or mist with cooking spray. Bake for 25 to 30 minutes, until the cauliflower florets are golden brown and crispy. Serve hot with the ranch dressing.

CHAPTER 20

A Little Something on the Side-Side Dishes

Sometimes you just need a little somethin'-somethin' on the side. You know, to help round things out, or to fill a void. Or, when it comes to meals, an empty place on your plate that needs to be filled up with a tasty side dish or two. This chapter has a whole slew of bean, grain, and veggie-based side dish selections, all of which are made either in the oven or on the stove top.

Citrus-Scented Asparagus

MAKES 2 SERVINGS

There is something so sensual about eating with your fingers! Many people prefer to eat whole asparagus spears with their fingers, rather than a fork, and if that's your preference, then only cook these lemony ones until crisp-tender.

- 1 pound asparagus, ends trimmed
- 1½ teaspoons olive oil, or 1 to 2 tablespoons water
- 1 tablespoon minced garlic
- Zest and juice of 1 lemon
- 2 tablespoon chopped fresh parsley
- Sea salt
- Freshly ground black pepper

1. Put the asparagus and oil in a large cast-iron or nonstick skillet and cook over medium heat, stirring occasionally, for 3 minutes.

2. Add the garlic, lemon zest and juice, and parsley and cook, stirring occasionally, for 2 to 3 minutes, until desired tenderness. Season with salt and pepper to taste. Serve hot.

Variation: For an oil-free version, replace the olive oil with 2 to 3 tablespoons water or vegetable broth. For a spicy version, sprinkle crushed red pepper flakes over the finished dish.

Lemon and Ginger-Infused Steamed Vegetables

MAKES 4 SERVINGS

One of the healthiest ways to cook vegetables is by steaming them until they're crisp-tender. Adding half a lemon and some slices of ginger to the cooking water will subtly infuse their flavors into the vegetables. Serve them up as is, or alongside your favorite dipping sauce.

- 1 lemon, cut in half
- 1 (1-inch) piece fresh ginger, thinly sliced
- 1½ cups small broccoli florets
- 1½ cups small cauliflower florets
- 1 cup halved baby carrots, or 1 cup carrots, cut diagonally into ¼-inch thick slices
- 1 cup asparagus, ends trimmed and cut in half diagonally
- 1 cup snap peas or pea pods
- Sea salt
- Freshly ground black pepper or lemon pepper

1. Leave one half of the lemon intact, and then cut the other half into 4 wedges and set aside.

2. Set up a large pot with a collapsible steamer basket or steamer rack insert. Add enough water so that it just touches the bottom of the collapsible steamer, or 2 inches deep if using a rack insert. Put the intact lemon half and ginger slices into the water. Cover the pot and bring to a boil over medium heat.

3. In batches, steam the vegetables, until crisp-tender - broccoli and cauliflower for 5 to 7 minutes, carrots for 3 to 5 minutes, and asparagus and snap peas for 2 to 3 minutes.

4. Transfer the steamed vegetables to a large bowl and stir to combine. Alternatively, arrange the vegetables in rows or in a circle on a large plate or platter. Season with salt and pepper to taste.

5.   Squeeze the juice of one lemon wedge over each serving as desired. Serve hot or at room temperature, either plain, or with Creamy Hemp Seed Dressing (see Cleopatra Salad with Hemp Seed Dressing in Afternoon Delights), Cheesy Sauce (see Bacon Cheeseburger Mac-n-Cheese in Main Events), or Creamy Saffron-Almond Dipping Sauce (see Steamed Artichokes with Creamy Saffron-Almond Dipping Sauce in this chapter).

Steamed Artichokes with Creamy Saffron-Almond Dipping Sauce

MAKES 4 SERVINGS (1 ARTICHOKE AND
¼ CUP SAFFRON-ALMOND DIPPING SAUCE)

At first, you may be a bit intimidated about how to approach eating a whole artichoke, but it's really quite easy, and it can be a very sensual experience! Here's what you do: one-at-a-time, peel off the outer petal-like leaves, dip the white fleshy end of the leaf into your favorite dipping sauce (or not), then place that portion upside-down in your mouth, clamp down on it with your teeth, and then pull it through your teeth to remove and enjoy the soft fleshy portion. Continue eating all of the leaves, in this manner, until you reach the inner artichoke heart. With a knife or spoon, scrape off the inedible, fuzzy top part (called the choke), discard it, and the artichoke heart will be revealed, which you can (and should) eat as well. There you have it, and hopefully, you and your lover will have fun eating these steamed artichokes and their saffron-infused dipping sauce.

- 4 large whole artichokes
- 1 lemon, cut in half

Creamy Saffron-Almond Dipping Sauce:
- 3 tablespoons hot water
- Pinch of saffron threads
- 1 medium shallot, finely diced, or ½ cup finely diced yellow onion

- ¼ cup raw sliced almonds
- 2 large cloves garlic
- 1½ tablespoons lemon juice
- 1 cup plain nondairy yogurt
- Sea salt
- Freshly ground black pepper

---

1. To prep each artichoke for steaming, (pulling downward toward the stem) snap off a few of the tough outer leaves and discard. Using a serrated knife, cut off the bottom stem, and then cut a little off the top (about 1 inch) and discard. Using kitchen scissors, snip off the sharp thorny tips and discard. Rub the cut surfaces of the artichoke with half of a lemon to prevent discoloration. Repeat the procedure for the remaining artichokes.

2. Set up a large pot with a collapsible steamer basket or steamer rack insert. Add enough water so that it just touches the bottom of the collapsible steamer, or 2 inches deep if using a rack insert. Put the lemon halves in the water. Cover the pot and bring to a boil over medium heat.

3. Put the artichokes in the steamer and steam for 25 to 35 minutes, until the inner artichoke hearts are easily pierced with the tip of a knife and the inner leaves pull out easily. Remove the artichokes from the steamer and place them on a large plate or platter.

4. While the artichokes are steaming, prepare the saffron-almond dipping sauce. Put 1 tablespoon of hot water and saffron in a small bowl. Let sit for 10 minutes to soften the saffron.

5. Put the remaining 2 tablespoon of hot water, shallot, almonds, and garlic in a small saucepan and cook over medium heat, stirring occasionally, for 3 to 5 minutes, until the shallot is tender and all of the water has evaporated.

6. Transfer the shallot mixture to a food processor. Add the saffron mixture and lemon juice and process until smooth. Add the yogurt and process for 30 seconds. Season with salt and pepper to taste and process for 15 seconds. Serve hot or at room temperature as desired, each artichoke with ¼ cup of the saffron-almond dipping sauce in a small bowl.

Variation: If you can't find (or can't afford) saffron, replace it with a pinch of ground turmeric, but don't soak it in water, and instead add it directly to the blender. Or, you can skip making the dipping sauce altogether, and instead, serve the artichokes with a side of melted vegan butter.

Roman-Style Artichoke and Asparagus Bake

MAKES 4 SERVINGS

Without a doubt, Rome is one of the most romantic cities in Italy, and it provided the inspiration for this quick-and-easy, oven-baked side dish. Artichokes, asparagus, basil, garlic, olives, and tomatoes are all commonly used ingredients in Italian cuisine, and their colors and flavors complement each other deliciously in this flavorful casserole.

- 1 pound asparagus, ends trimmed and cut diagonally into 2-inch pieces
- 1 can (14 ounces) artichoke hearts packed in water, drained and each heart quartered
- 1½ cups diced tomatoes
- ¾ cup pitted black olives (preferably Kalamata olives), each olive quartered lengthwise
- ½ cup chopped fresh basil, lightly packed
- 1½ tablespoons minced garlic
- 1 tablespoon nutritional yeast flakes
- ½ teaspoon crushed red pepper flakes
- ½ teaspoon sea salt
- ¼ teaspoon freshly ground black pepper

1. Preheat the oven to 425 degrees F. Lightly oil a 9-inch baking pan or mist it with cooking spray.

2. Put all of the ingredients in a large bowl and stir to combine. Transfer the vegetable mixture to the oiled baking pan.

3. Bake for 7 minutes. Remove from the oven. Stir the vegetable mixture. Bake for 5 to 10 minutes longer, until the vegetables are tender. Serve hot.

Broccoli and Cheese-Topped Baked Potatoes

MAKES 4 SERVINGS

Transform your plain baked potatoes from ho-hum to yum by topping them with some cheesy sauce and cooked broccoli florets. Yes, it's that easy, plus you can make the cheesy-tasting sauce while the potatoes are baking in the oven (or cooking in the microwave). Serve them as a tasty side dish, or pair them with a salad for a filling lunch or dinner option.

- 4 large Russet potatoes
- Sea salt
- Freshly ground black pepper
- 2 cups small broccoli florets
- 1 recipe Cheesy Sauce (see Bacon Cheeseburger Mac-n-Cheese in Main Events)

1. To cook the potatoes in the oven, preheat the oven to 400 degrees F. Line a baking sheet with parchment paper or a silicone baking mat. Using a fork, pierce each potato in several places on all sides, and place them on the lined baking sheet. Bake for 40 to 45 minutes (flipping them over after 25 minutes), until the potatoes are soft and can be easily squeezed.

2. Alternatively, to cook the pierced potatoes in the microwave, place them in a pie pan or baking dish, and microwave for 15 to 20 minutes, until the potatoes are soft.

3. Using a sharp knife, cut a slit down the length of each potato, then gently squeeze to open, and place them on a large platter or on individual plates. Alternatively, cut each potato in half lengthwise, and place them, cut-side-up on a platter or plate. Season each potato with salt and pepper to taste.

4. Cook the broccoli florets by either steaming, microwaving, or boiling in them water until desired tenderness.

5. Top each potato with ⅓ to ½ cup cheesy sauce as desired and ½ cup cooked broccoli florets. Serve hot.

Variation: For added flavor and texture, also top each potato with 1 slice Tempeh Bacon (see recipe in Lingering Breakfasts (or Brunches) in Bed), coarsely chopped, or 1 tablespoon Coconut Bacon (see Avocado Toast with Coconut Bacon in Morning Quickies).

Ginger and Coconut
Water-Braised Carrots

MAKES 4 SERVINGS

When you slowly cook foods in a tightly covered pot with a small amount of liquid (like broth, water, or wine), that's called braising. In this case, carrots and grated fresh ginger are braised in coconut water, and then finished with a little chopped parsley and your choice of coconut oil or vegan butter.

- 1 pound carrots, cut in half lengthwise and cut into 2-inch pieces, or 1 pound whole baby carrots
- ⅔ cup coconut water
- 1½ tablespoons peeled and grated fresh ginger
- ⅓ cup chopped fresh parsley, lightly packed
- 1½ teaspoons coconut oil or nonhydrogenated vegan butter (optional)
- Sea salt

1. Put the carrots, coconut water, and ginger in a large saucepan. Cover and cook over medium heat for 10 to 12 minutes, until the carrots are tender.

2. Add the parsley and optional coconut oil and stir to combine. Season with salt to taste. Serve hot.

Variation: For a richer-tasting dish, replace the coconut water with ⅔ cup plain coconut milk beverage or canned coconut milk.

Ginger and Maple-Candied Carrots: After cooking the carrots until tender, add 2 tablespoons maple syrup to the saucepan, and cook uncovered, stirring occasionally, for 2 to 3 minutes, until the cooking liquid thickens to a glaze-like consistency.

Spiced and Smashed Sweet Potatoes

MAKES 4 SERVINGS

Cooked sweet potatoes are mashed with sweet maple syrup, coconut oil, cinnamon, nutmeg, and vanilla, plus a shot of bourbon, to create this swoon-worthy side dish. Serve them straight up, or top them with one or more of the suggested garnishes.

- 1½ pounds (4 to 5 medium) sweet potatoes, peeled and cut into 2-inch cubes
- 2 tablespoons maple syrup
- 2 tablespoons bourbon
- 2 teaspoons coconut oil or nonhydrogenated vegan butter (optional)
- 1½ teaspoons ground cinnamon
- 1 teaspoon vanilla extract
- ¼ teaspoon freshly grated nutmeg
- Garnish options: ⅓ cup toasted and coarsely chopped pecans or pumpkin seeds, or ¼ cup toasted unsweetened shredded dried coconut

1. Put the sweet potatoes in a large saucepan or soup pot and cover with water. Cook over medium-high heat for 20 to 25 minutes, until the sweet potatoes are tender. Reserve ⅓ cup of the cooking water. Drain the sweet potatoes in a colander.

2. Put the reserved cooking water back into the saucepan. Add the maple syrup, bourbon, optional coconut oil, cinnamon, vanilla extract, and nutmeg and stir to combine. Bring to a boil over medium heat. Remove from the heat.

3. Add the sweet potatoes to the saucepan. Using a potato masher, mash the sweet potatoes until smooth and creamy. Top the sweet potato mixture with one or more of the suggested garnishes as desired. Serve hot.

Bayou Beans

MAKES 4 SERVINGS

Down in New Orleans they often cook their beans with sausage, much like this spicy batch of beans that are made with seitan sausages. Also making an appearance is the "holy trinity" of Cajun cooking--onion, celery, and bell pepper. For a real down-home meal, serve the beans over cornbread or cooked rice.

- 1 cup dried red beans or kidney beans, sorted and rinsed
- ⅔ cup diced yellow onion
- ⅔ cup diced celery
- ⅔ cup diced red or green bell pepper
- 1 tablespoon olive oil, or ¼ cup low-sodium vegetable broth or water
- 1 jalapeño chile, seeded and finely diced
- 1½ tablespoons minced garlic
- 1½ teaspoons chili powder
- 1 teaspoon dried oregano
- 1 teaspoon dried thyme
- ¼ teaspoon cayenne or chipotle chili powder
- 3½ cups water
- 1 bay leaf
- 3 Seitan Sausages (see recipe in Lingering Breakfasts (or Brunches) in Bed), coarsely chopped
- ⅓ cup thinly sliced green onions
- Sea salt
- Freshly ground black pepper

1. Put the red beans in a large saucepan or soup pot and cover with warm water. Let soak for several hours or overnight. Drain the red beans in a colander and set aside. Rinse the saucepan (or soup pot) and reuse.

2. Put the onion, celery, bell pepper, and oil (for an oil-free version use vegetable broth) in the large saucepan (or soup pot) and cook over medium heat, stirring occasionally, for 5 minutes.

3. Add the jalapeño chile, garlic, chili powder, oregano, thyme, and cayenne and cook, stirring occasionally, for 2 minutes.

4. Add the beans, water, and bay leaf and stir to combine. Bring to a boil over high heat. Cover, decrease the heat to low, and simmer for 1 hour, until the red beans are soft.

5. Remove the bay leaf and discard. Add the seitan sausages and green onions and cook, stirring occasionally, for 5 minutes. Season with salt and pepper to taste. Serve hot.

Okra Soycutash

MAKES 4 SERVINGS

In this revamped, deep South-inspired version of a traditional succotash recipe, lima beans are replaced with plump shelled edamame. To further change things up, a jalapeño chile and frozen sliced okra are added to the traditional mix of corn, bell pepper, and tomatoes.

- 1 package (10 ounces) frozen cut corn
- 1 package (10 ounces) frozen sliced okra
- 1 cup diced red bell pepper
- ⅔ cup diced tomatoes
- ⅔ cup frozen shelled edamame
- ½ cup low-sodium vegetable broth
- 1 jalapeño chile, cut in half lengthwise and thinly sliced
- ⅓ cup thinly sliced green onions
- ¼ cup chopped fresh parsley, lightly packed
- 1 tablespoon nutritional yeast flakes
- 1 teaspoon chili powder
- 1 teaspoon dried oregano
- 1 teaspoon dried thyme
- ¼ teaspoon cayenne or chipotle chile powder
- Sea salt
- Freshly ground black pepper

1. Put the corn, okra, bell pepper, tomatoes, edamame, vegetable broth, and jalapeño chile in a large pot or nonstick skillet and stir to combine. Cover and cook over medium-high heat, stirring occasionally, for 8 to 10 minutes, until the vegetables are tender.

2. Add the green onions, parsley, nutritional yeast, chili powder, oregano, thyme, and cayenne and cook uncovered, stirring occasionally, for 1 to 2 minutes, until the broth has evaporated. Season with salt and pepper to taste. Serve hot.

Roasted Roots

MAKES 4 SERVINGS

Undoubtedly, root vegetables have an "earthy" flavor because they grow deep within the dirt, but there's a bit of sweetness hidden within their depths as well. You can easily help your root vegetables to release their natural sugars by oven-roasting them. For this recipe, beets are paired with another root vegetable of your choosing, roasted with a covering of herbs, vegetable broth, and olive oil, and then given a balsamic vinegar finish.

- 1 pound beets
- 1 pound root vegetables of choice (such as rutabagas, turnips, or parsnips or a combination)
- ¼ cup low-sodium vegetable broth
- 1½ tablespoons olive oil
- 1 tablespoon nutritional yeast flakes
- 4 large cloves garlic, thinly sliced
- 2 teaspoons Italian seasonings blend, or ½ teaspoon each dried basil, oregano, and rosemary
- Sea salt
- Freshly ground black pepper
- 2 tablespoons balsamic vinegar

1. Preheat the oven to 400 degrees F. Line a baking sheet with parchment paper or a silicone baking mat.

2. Peel the beets and root vegetables if desired, and then cut them into 1½-inch cubes or small wedges.

3. Put the vegetable broth, oil, nutritional yeast, garlic, and Italian seasonings blend in a large bowl and whisk to combine. Add the cut beets and root vegetables and stir to evenly coat them with the broth mixture. Transfer the mixture to the lined baking sheet and spread them into a single layer.

4. Bake for 20 minutes. Remove from the oven. Stir the mixture with a metal spatula and spread into a single layer again. Bake for 15 to 20

minutes longer, until the vegetables are tender and lightly browned around the edges.

5.   Remove from the oven. Season with salt and pepper to taste. Drizzle the balsamic vinegar over the top of the vegetables and stir with a metal spatula to combine. Serve hot.

Tomatoes Rockefeller

MAKES 4 SERVINGS

Oysters Rockefeller, named for millionaire John D. Rockefeller, was created at Antoine's Restaurant in New Orleans back in 1899. It was named as such because the unfortunate oysters on the half shell were topped with a rich, buttery-tasting and green-tinted (like money) topping. For this veganized version, large tomato halves are used to hold a spinach-based filling that's topped with breadcrumbs.

- 2 large tomatoes
- ½ cup finely diced yellow onion, or 1 medium shallot, finely diced
- 1 tablespoon olive oil, or 2 to 3 tablespoons low-sodium vegetable broth or water
- 4 cups coarsely chopped baby spinach, lightly packed
- 1½ tablespoons minced garlic
- ¼ cup chopped fresh basil, lightly packed
- 2 tablespoons chopped fresh parsley
- 1 tablespoon nutritional yeast flakes
- ¼ teaspoon smoked or sweet paprika
- ¼ teaspoon sea salt
- ⅛ teaspoon freshly ground black pepper
- ⅛ teaspoon freshly grated nutmeg
- 2 tablespoons dry or fresh breadcrumbs

1. Preheat the oven to 375 degrees F.

2. To prep the tomatoes, cut each tomato in half crosswise. Using your fingers, gently remove the seeds from each tomato half (you want to keep the tomato half intact) and discard the seeds. Place the tomato halves cut-side-up and side-by-side in a baking dish.

3. Put the onion and oil (for an oil-free version use vegetable broth) in a large cast iron or nonstick skillet and cook over medium heat, stirring occasionally, for 3 minutes.

4. Add the spinach and garlic and cook, stirring occasionally, for 2 to 3 minutes, until the spinach is wilted. Add the basil, parsley, nutritional

yeast, paprika, salt, pepper, and nutmeg and stir to combine. Remove from the heat.

5. Evenly dividing, place the spinach mixture on top of each tomato half. Sprinkle ½ tablespoon of breadcrumbs over the top of each tomato half.

6. Bake for 15 to 20 minutes, until the tomatoes are slightly soft and the breadcrumbs are lightly browned. Serve hot.

Pistachio and Grape-Studded Quinoa

MAKES 4 SERVINGS

Not all side dishes have to be savory and served up hot. On the contrary, their flavor can be more on the sweet side, and they can served warm, at room temperature, or even cold and still be quite pleasing. Like this one, in which cooked quinoa is first cloaked with a toasted sesame oil and cinnamon-infused dressing mixture, and then studded with juicy red and white grapes, cucumber pieces, and pistachios.

- 1 cup white, red, or tri-color quinoa, rinsed
- ¾ cup apple juice
- ⅔ cup water
- 1 tablespoon peeled and grated fresh ginger
- 2 tablespoons red wine vinegar or apple cider vinegar
- 1 tablespoon toasted sesame oil
- 1 teaspoon agave nectar or maple syrup
- ½ teaspoon sea salt
- ¼ teaspoon freshly ground black pepper
- ¼ teaspoon ground cinnamon
- ½ cup diced cucumber
- ½ cup halved red seedless grapes
- ½ cup halved white seedless grapes
- ½ cup raw or roasted pistachios
- ¼ cup thinly sliced green onions
- ¼ cup chopped fresh parsley, lightly packed

1. Put the quinoa, apple juice, water, and ginger in medium saucepan and stir to combine. Bring to a boil over high heat. Cover, decrease the heat to low, and simmer for 15 to 18 minutes, until the quinoa is tender and all of the cooking liquid is absorbed.

2. Fluff the quinoa with a fork to loosen the grains. Let the quinoa cool for 10 minutes and then fluff the quinoa again. Transfer the quinoa to a large bowl.

3. To make the dressing mixture, put the vinegar, oil, agave nectar, salt, pepper, and cinnamon in a small bowl and whisk to combine. Pour the

dressing mixture over the quinoa and gently stir to evenly coat the quinoa.

4.   Add the cucumber, both seedless grapes, pistachios, green onions, and parsley and gently stir to combine. Serve warm, at room temperature, or cold as desired.

Variation: If you want, you can also serve this as a salad. Simply, double the amount of the dressing mixture, add 2 cups baby mixed greens or coarsely chopped leafy greens, and toss gently to combine.

Orange-Scented Couscous with Apricots, Cherries, and Pine Nuts

MAKES 4 SERVINGS

Lightly perfume your couscous with a hint of orange, simply by adding the zest and juice of a large one into the cooking water. To add a pop of color and textural contrast to the beige-colored couscous, combine with some vibrantly-pink pickled onions, toasted pine nuts, and chewy pieces of dried apricots and cherries.

- 1 cup water
- Zest and juice of 1 orange (approximately 3 tablespoons zest and ½ cup juice)
- 1 tablespoon peeled and grated fresh ginger
- 1 cup white or whole wheat couscous
- 1½ tablespoons white wine or red wine vinegar
- 1 tablespoon olive oil
- ½ cup diced red onion
- ⅓ cup toasted pine nuts
- ⅓ cup coarsely chopped dried apricots
- ⅓ cup dried cherries or dried cranberries
- ⅓ cup chopped fresh parsley, lightly packed
- Sea salt
- Freshly ground black pepper

1. Put the water, orange zest and juice, and ginger in a medium saucepan. Bring to a boil over high heat. Add the couscous. Cover and remove from the heat. Let sit for 5 minutes to allow the couscous to absorb the liquid.

2. Fluff the couscous with a fork to loosen the grains. Add 1 tablespoon of vinegar and oil and gently stir to evenly coat the couscous.

3. Rinse out the saucepan and reuse. Fill the saucepan with 1 inch of water. Bring to a boil over high heat. Add the onion and boil for 30 seconds. Drain the onion in a colander and return the onion to the saucepan. Add the remaining ½ tablespoon of vinegar and stir to combine (this will turn the onion a vibrant pink color).

4. To the couscous mixture, add the onion, pine nuts, apricots, cherries, and parsley and gently stir to combine. Season with salt and pepper to taste. Serve warm, at room temperature, or cold as desired.

Confetti Coconut Basmati Rice

MAKES 4 SERVINGS

To add a lot of exotic flavor and bit of creaminess, cooked basmati rice is combined with coconut milk, citrus juice, garlic, ginger, and red pepper flakes. After that, the coconut rice is embellished with black beans, red and orange bell peppers, green onions, and cilantro, and garnished with toasted coconut and almonds.

- 2 cups water
- 1 cup white or brown basmati rice, rinsed
- ¼ cup plain coconut milk beverage or canned coconut milk
- Juice of ½ a orange
- Juice of 1 lime
- 1 tablespoon minced garlic
- 1 tablespoon peeled and grated fresh ginger
- 1½ teaspoons toasted sesame oil or melted coconut oil
- ¼ teaspoon crushed red pepper flakes
- 1 can (15 ounces) black beans, drained and rinsed
- ½ cup diced orange or yellow bell pepper
- ½ cup diced red bell pepper
- ¼ cup thinly sliced green onions
- ¼ cup chopped fresh cilantro or parsley, lightly packed
- Sea salt
- Freshly ground black pepper
- ¼ cup toasted unsweetened coconut chips, or 2 tablespoons toasted unsweetened shredded dried coconut

1. Put the water and rice in a medium saucepan. Bring to a boil over high heat. Cover, decrease the heat to low, and simmer for 20 minutes (for white basmati) to 30 minutes (for brown basmati), until the rice is tender and all of the water is absorbed. Remove from the heat.

2. Fluff the rice with a fork to loosen the grains. Add the milk, orange juice, lime juice, garlic, ginger, oil, and red pepper flakes and gently stir to combine.

3. Add the black beans, both bell peppers, green onions, and cilantro and gently stir to combine. Season with salt and pepper to taste. Scatter the toasted coconut over the top. Serve hot, warm, or at room temperature as desired.

Down-n-Dirty Rice

MAKES 4 SERVINGS

Dirty rice is a Cajun rice dish that's traditionally made with spices, aromatic vegetables, and chopped chicken livers. This meatless version contains many of the traditional components, as well as a mixture of coarsely chopped and pan-cooked mushrooms, nuts, and sunflower seeds, used to create a similar consistency and savory flavor.

- 2 cups water
- 1 cup mixed rice and wild rice blend or long-grain brown rice, rinsed
- ½ cup raw nuts (such as almonds, pecans, walnuts, or a combination), coarsely chopped
- 2 tablespoons raw sunflower seeds, coarsely chopped
- 1 cup finely diced button or cremini mushrooms
- ½ cup finely diced yellow onion
- ½ cup finely diced celery
- 2 teaspoons olive oil, or ¼ cup low-sodium vegetable broth
- ¼ cup thinly sliced green onions
- 2 tablespoons minced garlic
- 1½ teaspoons chili powder
- 1½ teaspoons dried oregano
- 1½ teaspoons dried thyme
- ¼ teaspoon freshly ground black pepper
- ¼ teaspoon cayenne or hot pepper sauce
- ⅓ cup chopped fresh parsley, lightly packed
- 1½ tablespoons reduced-sodium tamari or coconut aminos

1. Put the water and rice in a medium saucepan. Bring to a boil over high heat. Cover, decrease the heat to low, and simmer for 35 to 40 minutes, until the rice is tender and all of the water is absorbed. Remove from the heat.

2. While the rice is cooking, put the nuts and sunflower seeds in a (dry) large cast iron or nonstick skillet and cook over medium heat, stirring occasionally, for 3 to 5 minutes, until the nut mixture is lightly toasted and fragrant. Transfer the nut mixture to a small plate and set aside.

3. Rinse the skillet and reuse. Put the mushrooms, onion, celery, and oil (for an oil-free version use vegetable broth) in the skillet and cook over medium-high heat, stirring occasionally, for 5 minutes. Add the green onions, garlic, chili powder, oregano, thyme, pepper, and cayenne and cook, stirring occasionally, for 2 to 3 minutes, until the vegetables are tender. Remove from the heat.

4. Fluff the rice with a fork to loosen the grains. To the vegetable mixture, add the rice, reserved nut mixture, parsley, and tamari and stir to combine. Serve hot.

Down-n-Dirty Cauliflower Rice: Replace the cooked rice with 3 cups (store-bought) cauliflower rice. Alternatively, transform 1 medium head of cauliflower into small, rice-like pieces either using a food processor or grate by hand with a box grater.

Farro with Lacinato Kale and Pomegranate Seeds

MAKES 4 SERVINGS

Farro is considered by many to be the mother of all wheat species, and it was a staple in the daily diet of ancient Rome. To honor its Italian roots, farro is paired with cooked lacinato kale, red onion, garlic, raisins, pomegranate seeds, and toasted almonds.

- 3 cups water
- 1 cup farro, rinsed
- 1 bunch lacinato kale, stemmed and cut into thin ribbons
- ½ cup diced red onion
- 1 tablespoon olive oil, or 2 to 3 tablespoons water
- 1 tablespoon minced garlic
- ½ cup chopped fresh parsley, lightly packed
- ⅓ cup raisins (preferably golden raisins)
- Juice of ½ a lemon
- ⅓ cup pomegranate seeds
- ⅓ cup toasted sliced almonds
- Sea salt
- Freshly ground black pepper

1. Put the water and farro in a medium saucepan. Bring to a boil over high heat. Cover, decrease the heat to low, and simmer for 30 to 40 minutes, until the farro is tender and all of the water is absorbed. Remove from the heat.

2. While the farro is cooking, put the kale, red onion, and oil (for an oil-free version use water) in a large cast iron or nonstick skillet and cook over medium-high heat, stirring occasionally, for 5 minutes. Add the garlic and cook, stirring occasionally, for 2 to 3 minutes, until the kale is tender. Remove from the heat.

3. Add the farro, raisins, parsley, and lemon juice and stir to combine. Season with salt and pepper to taste. Add the pomegranate seeds and almonds and stir to combine. Serve hot or at room temperature as desired.

Variation: If you can't find farro, you can replace it with 1 cup wheat berries or spelt berries, but increase the cooking time to 1 hour or until they're tender.

CHAPTER 21

Main Events–Main Dishes

What's for dinner? We've all heard (or wondered about) that one hundreds, if not thousands, of times when our loved one(s) come sauntering through the door. In other words, people are hungry in the house and you need to get the food on the table fast! All of these main dish recipes are healthy and filling. If you're pressed for time, then you'll really appreciate the quick-cooking recipes, but most of the recipes in this chapter are ready in under an hour anyway. Plus, they're varied enough to appeal to a wide variety of tastes, from finicky eaters to those with big appetites. So, whether you're feeding a family of four, or there's a chance that you and your lover may want seconds, don't worry, there will be enough to go around because all of the recipes in this chapter make enough for four servings.

Mushroom and Veggie Fajitas

MAKES 4 SERVINGS

To make these fabulous fajitas, a mixture of thickly sliced mushrooms, onions, and bell peppers are cloaked with a zesty lime dressing, then left to marinate for a bit, before being cooked up in a skillet. The cooked vegetables are then folded up in flour tortillas with sliced avocado and diced tomatoes.

- Zest and juice of 2 limes
- 2 tablespoons minced garlic
- 1½ tablespoons olive oil
- 1 teaspoon dried oregano
- 1 teaspoon chili powder, or ½ teaspoon chipotle chile powder and ¼ teaspoon crushed red pepper flakes
- 2 portobello mushrooms, halved and cut into ½-inch thick slices, or 2½ cups sliced button or cremini mushrooms
- 1 large red or yellow onion, cut into ½-inch thick slices
- 1 medium green pepper, cut into ½-inch thick slices
- 1 medium orange or red bell pepper, cut into ½-inch thick slices
- 1 jalapeño chile, seeded and finely diced (optional)
- ⅓ cup chopped fresh cilantro, lightly packed
- Sea salt
- Freshly ground black pepper
- 4 (8-inch or larger) flour tortillas
- 1 avocado, thinly sliced
- 1 cup diced tomatoes

1. Put the lime zest and juice, garlic, oil, oregano, and chili powder in a large bowl and stir to combine.

2. Add the mushrooms, onion, both bell peppers, optional jalapeño chile, and cilantro and stir to combine. Season with salt and pepper to taste. Let the vegetable mixture sit for 10 minutes to marinate.

3. Put the marinated vegetable mixture in a large cast iron or nonstick skillet and cook over medium-high heat, stirring occasionally, for 8 to 10 minutes, until the vegetables are tender.

4. To assemble the fajitas, place each tortilla on a large plate. Evenly dividing, place one-quarter of the vegetable mixture horizontally in the center of each tortilla. Top each fajita with one-quarter of the sliced avocado and ¼ cup diced tomatoes. Serve hot.

Green Gumbo

MAKES 4 SERVINGS

Green gumbo (or gumbo z'herbes) is a hearty stew made with a generous amount of leafy greens, onion, celery, bell pepper, and jalapeño chiles. As a plus, this vegan version features chewy spiced mushrooms as a replacement for the commonly used andouille sausage. Enjoy bowlfuls of this gumbo with or without cooked rice or other grains on top.

- ¼ cup whole wheat flour or unbleached all-purpose flour
- 2 tablespoons olive oil, or ¼ to ⅓ cup low-sodium vegetable broth
- 1 cup diced green bell pepper
- 1 cup diced celery
- 1 cup diced yellow onion
- 2 jalapeño chiles, seeded and finely diced
- 2 tablespoons minced garlic
- 2 bunches leafy greens (any combination of collard greens, kale, mustard greens, turnips greens, Swiss chard, or spinach), stemmed and cut into thin strips
- 3½ cups water
- 2 cups shredded green cabbage, lightly packed
- 1 bay leaf
- 6 ounces (about 3 cups) coarsely chopped button or cremini mushrooms
- 1 tablespoon chili powder
- 1 teaspoon dried oregano
- 1 teaspoon dried thyme
- 2 tablespoons nutritional yeast flakes
- ¼ cup chopped fresh parsley, lightly packed
- Sea salt
- Freshly ground black pepper

1. Put the flour and 1½ tablespoons of oil (for an oil-free version use vegetable broth) in a large soup pot and cook over medium heat, stirring occasionally, for 10 to 12 minutes, until golden brown.

2. Add the bell pepper, celery, onion, jalapeño chiles, and garlic and cook, stirring occasionally, for 5 to 7 minutes, until the vegetables are soft.

3. Add the leafy greens, water, cabbage, and bay leaf and stir to combine. Bring to a boil over high heat. Cover, decrease the heat to low, and simmer for 25 minutes.

4. While the vegetable mixture is simmering, put the mushrooms and remaining ½ tablespoon of oil in a large cast iron or nonstick skillet and cook over medium-high heat, stirring occasionally, for 7 to 8 minutes, until lightly browned. Add the chili powder, oregano, and thyme and cook, stirring occasionally, for 2 minutes.

5. To the soup pot mixture, add the mushroom mixture, nutritional yeast, and parsley and simmer, stirring occasionally, for 5 minutes longer. Remove the bay leaf and discard. Season with salt and pepper to taste. Serve hot, either plain or topped with cooked brown rice or grains as desired.

Veggie Paella

MAKES 4 SERVINGS

Spain is famous for its Paella, which is a saffron-infused rice dish that's made with an assortment of seafood and vegetables. For this veganized version, the seafood is left in the sea, and instead features a colorful blend of mushrooms, artichokes, red bell pepper, peas, tomatoes, and olives.

- 2 cups low-sodium vegetable broth
- ½ teaspoon sea salt
- ¼ teaspoon freshly ground black pepper
- ¼ teaspoon saffron threads or ground turmeric
- ⅔ cup halved and thinly sliced button or cremini mushrooms
- ½ cup diced yellow onion
- ½ cup diced red bell pepper
- 1½ tablespoons olive oil
- 1 cup long-grain white rice, rinsed
- ½ cup diced tomatoes
- 1 tablespoon minced garlic
- ½ cup artichoke hearts, each heart quartered
- ½ cup frozen peas (thawed), or ½ cup pea pods, cut in half diagonally
- ⅓ cup pitted Kalamata olives or other black olives, sliced
- ¼ cup chopped fresh parsley, lightly packed
- 1 tablespoon lemon juice

1. Put the vegetable broth, salt, pepper, and saffron in a small saucepan and bring to a simmer over low heat.

2. Put the mushrooms, onion, bell pepper, and oil in a large cast-iron or nonstick skillet and cook over medium heat, stirring occasionally, for 5 minutes. Add the rice and stir to evenly coat the rice with the oil. Add the tomato, and garlic and cook, stirring constantly, for 2 minutes.

3. Add the simmering broth to the rice mixture and stir to combine. Bring to a boil over high heat. Cover, decrease the heat to low, and simmer for 15 to 20 minutes, until the rice is tender and all of the water is absorbed. Remove from the heat.

4. Fluff the rice with a fork to loosen the grains. Add the artichokes, peas, olives, parsley, and lemon juice and stir to combine. Serve hot.

Sweet and Sour Tofu and Vegetables
MAKES 4 SERVINGS

Our tongues are designed to appreciate the contrast of sweet and sour flavors, and these two opposing tastes are often culinary mates. Like in this Chinese take-out favorite, which features large pieces of tofu, carrots, celery, bell pepper, broccoli, red onion, and pineapple chunks. This tofu-and-veggie combo is then covered with a sweet, sour, and slightly tangy sauce. Serve over cooked rice or grains.

Sweet and Sour Sauce:
- 1 can (15 ounces) pineapple chunks
- 2 tablespoons ketchup
- 2 tablespoons reduced-sodium tamari or coconut aminos
- 2 tablespoons brown rice vinegar or apple cider vinegar
- 2 tablespoons light brown sugar or coconut sugar
- 1 tablespoon minced ginger
- 1 tablespoon peeled and grated fresh ginger
- 1 tablespoon cornstarch

- 8 ounces firm or extra-firm tofu
- 2 teaspoons cornstarch
- 1 tablespoon sunflower oil or other oil
- 1½ cups small broccoli florets
- 2 medium carrots, thinly sliced diagonally
- 2 large stalks celery, thinly sliced diagonally
- 1 medium orange or red bell pepper, cut into 1-inch pieces
- ½ medium green bell pepper, cut into 1-inch pieces
- ½ small red onion, cut into half moons

1. To make the sweet and sour sauce, drain the juice from the can of pineapple chunks into a small bowl. Place the pineapple chunks on a small plate and set aside. Add the remaining sauce ingredients to the pineapple juice and whisk to combine.

2. To prep the tofu, squeeze the block of tofu over the sink to remove the excess water. Place the tofu in a colander in the sink, cover with a plate, place a heavy can (or other weight) on top of the plate, and let the tofu press for 20 minutes.

3. Transfer the pressed tofu to a cutting board and cut into 1-inch cubes. Place the tofu cubes on a large plate, sprinkle the cornstarch over the top, and gently toss until to evenly coat the tofu cubes on all sides.

4. Put the coated tofu cubes and oil in a large cast iron or nonstick skillet and cook over medium heat, stirring occasionally, for 10 to 12 minutes, until the tofu cubes are lightly browned on all sides. Using a slotted spoon, remove the tofu cubes from the skillet, and transfer to a large plate.

5. To the skillet, add the broccoli, carrots, celery, both bell peppers, and onion and cook, stirring occasionally, for 3 to 5 minutes, until the vegetables are crisp-tender. Add the reserved pineapple chunks and cook, stirring occasionally, for 1 minute.

6. Add the reserved tofu cubes and sweet and sour sauce and cook, stirring constantly, for 1 to 2 minutes, until the sauce thickens. Serve hot over cooked rice or grains.

Sweet and Sour Tempeh and Vegetables: Replace the tofu with 1 package (8 ounces) tempeh, cut into 1-inch cubes. You don't need to press the tempeh first.

Pesto-Swirled Polenta

MAKES 4 SERVINGS

If you've got some cornmeal in your pantry, then you can make a batch of polenta, which is an Italian comfort food that's filling and oh-so-affordable to prepare. This thick and creamy polenta is flavored with nutritional yeast and olive oil, and then finished with a decorative swirl of fresh herbed pesto.

Herb Pesto:
- 1½ cups fresh basil leaves, lightly packed
- 1 cup parsley leaves, lightly packed
- ¼ cup toasted pine nuts, or ⅓ cup toasted walnuts
- 2 tablespoons nutritional yeast flakes
- 1 tablespoon olive oil
- 1 tablespoon water
- 3 large cloves garlic
- ½ teaspoon sea salt
- ⅛ teaspoon freshly ground black pepper

Polenta:
- 6 cups water
- ¾ teaspoon sea salt
- ½ teaspoon freshly ground black pepper
- 1½ cups medium-grind or coarse cornmeal
- 2 tablespoon nutritional yeast flakes
- 1 tablespoon olive oil or nonhydrogenated vegan butter (optional)
- Crushed red pepper flakes (optional)

1. To make the herb pesto, put all of the ingredients in a food processor and process until smooth. Scrape down the sides of the container with a spatula and process for 15 seconds.

2. To make the polenta, put the water, salt, and pepper in a large saucepan. Bring to a boil over high heat. Decrease to the heat to medium. Slowly whisk in the cornmeal (to prevent lumps) and cook, whisking constantly, for 1 to 2 minutes, until the mixture begins to boil again.

3. Decrease the heat to low. Cover and simmer, stirring every 10 minutes with a long-handled spoon, for 30 to 35 minutes, until the polenta is very thick and begins to pull away from the sides of the saucepan. Remove from the heat.

4.   Add the nutritional yeast and optional oil and stir to combine. For each servings of polenta, randomly drop 2 tablespoons of the herb pesto over the top of the polenta, and then snake a knife through the two mixtures to achieve a swirl effect. Garnish each serving with optional red pepper flakes if desired. Serve hot.

Variation: For a heartier dish, top each serving with ⅓ cup Lemon-Herb Roasted Chickpeas (see recipe in Naughty Nibbles) or 1 coarsely chopped Seitan Sausage (see recipe in Lingering Breakfast (or Brunches) in Bed).

Bacon Cheeseburger Mac-n-Cheese

MAKES 4 SERVINGS

Mac-n-Cheese is a classic comfort food that's loved by many, and this cooked pasta and cheesy sauce combo can be prepared and augmented in numerous ways. This bacon cheeseburger-inspired version starts by covering cooked elbow macaroni with a cheesy-tasting sauce, and then combining it with your choice of tempeh bacon or coconut bacon. If you like your mac-n-cheese simply prepared, leave out the bacon.

Cheesy Sauce:
- 1½ cups water
- 1 medium carrot, diced
- ¼ cup raw cashews
- ¼ cup diced yellow onion
- ¼ cup diced orange or red bell pepper
- 2 large cloves garlic
- 3 tablespoons nutritional yeast flakes
- 2 teaspoon tapioca starch or cornstarch
- 1 teaspoon mellow miso or other miso of choice
- ½ teaspoon chili powder
- ½ teaspoon smoked or sweet paprika
- ½ teaspoon sea salt
- ¼ teaspoon freshly ground black pepper

- 8 ounces dry elbow macaroni
- 4 slices Tempeh Bacon (see recipe in Lingering Breakfasts (or Brunches) in Bed), coarsely chopped, or 1 recipe Coconut Bacon (see Avocado Toast with Coconut Bacon in Morning Quickies)
- Sea salt
- Freshly ground black pepper

1. To make the cheesy sauce, put the water, carrot, cashews, onion, bell pepper, and garlic in a medium sauce pan. Bring to a boil over high heat. Cover, decrease the heat to low, and simmer for 8 to 10 minutes, until the vegetables are soft. Remove from the heat. Let cool for 5 minutes.

2. Transfer the vegetable mixture to a blender. Add the nutritional yeast, tapioca starch, miso, chili powder, paprika, salt, and pepper and process until smooth. Scrape down the sides of the container with a spatula and process for 15 seconds.

330

3. Put the cheesy sauce back in the medium saucepan and cook over medium heat, whisking occasionally, for 3 to 5 minutes, until the sauce is very thick. Remove from the heat.

4. To cook the pasta, fill a large saucepan two-thirds full with water. Add a little salt to the water as desired. Bring to a boil over medium-high heat.

5. Add the elbow macaroni and cook, stirring occasionally, according to the package instructions or until tender. Drain the elbow macaroni in a colander and put it back the large saucepan.

6. Add the reserved cheesy sauce and stir to combine. Season with salt and pepper to taste. Scatter the tempeh bacon (or coconut bacon) over the top or stir in as desired. Serve hot.

Mushroom Cheeseburger Mac-n-Cheese: Replace the tempeh bacon (or coconut bacon) topping with 3 cups thinly sliced button or cremini mushrooms. Cook the mushrooms in a skillet with ¼ cup water or 1½ teaspoons olive until tender, and then stir them into the finished mac-n-cheese.

Pasta Primavera

MAKES 4 SERVINGS

Spring time has long been associated with fertility. This light-tasting pasta dish contains a colorful blend of fresh and frozen vegetables that are available during the spring months. The cooked pasta and vegetables are then cloaked with a simple sauce made of vegetable broth, white wine, lemon zest and juice, vegan butter, and fresh herbs.

- 8 ounces dry pasta of choice (such as farfalle, rotini, penne, or ziti)
- ¾ cup low-sodium vegetable broth
- 1 large carrot, cut in half lengthwise and thinly sliced diagonally
- 1 cup asparagus, ends trimmed and thinly sliced diagonally into 1-inch pieces
- 1 cup diced orange or yellow bell pepper
- 2 cups coarsely chopped baby spinach or arugula, lightly packed
- ½ cup frozen peas or fava beans (thawed)
- ½ cup thinly sliced green onions
- ¼ cup white wine of choice (such as Chardonnay or Reisling)
- ¼ cup chopped fresh basil, lightly packed, or 2 tablespoons chopped fresh dill
- ¼ cup chopped fresh parsley, lightly packed
- Zest and juice 1 lemon
- 1½ tablespoons nutritional yeast flakes
- 1 tablespoon nonhydrogenated vegan butter
- Sea salt
- Freshly ground black pepper
- Crushed red pepper flakes

1. To cook the pasta, fill a large saucepan or soup pot two-thirds full with water and add a little salt to the water if desired. Bring to a boil over medium-high heat.

2. Add the pasta and cook, stirring occasionally, according to the package instructions or until tender. Drain the pasta in a colander.

3. While the pasta is cooking, cook the vegetables. Put ½ cup of vegetable broth, carrot, asparagus, and bell pepper in a large cast-iron or nonstick skillet and cook over medium heat, stirring occasionally, for 5 minutes. Add the spinach, peas, and green onions and cook, stirring occasionally, for 2 to 3 minutes, until the vegetables are tender.

3. Add the remaining ¼ cup of vegetable broth, wine, basil, parsley, lemon zest and juice, nutritional yeast, and vegan butter and cook, stirring occasionally, for 1 minute longer to blend the flavors. Remove from the heat.

4. Add the cooked pasta and gently toss to combine. Season with salt, pepper, and red pepper flakes to taste. Serve hot.

Variation: For a grain-free option, replace the cooked pasta with 2 large zucchini that have been made into noodles with a spiralizer or vegetable peeler.

Pasta Puttanesca

MAKES 4 SERVINGS

The infamous Italian sauce, known as *puttanesca*, is named for the "ladies of the evening" because they could quickly prepare the sauce between their visitors, who were often lured by its aroma to their door. This spicy sauce is made with crushed tomatoes, onion, bell pepper, olives, capers, and fresh basil and parsley, and then tossed together with cooked spaghetti or linguine.

- 8 ounces dry spaghetti or linguine
- ⅔ cup diced yellow onion
- ⅔ cup diced red or green bell pepper
- 2 teaspoons olive oil, or ¼ cup low-sodium vegetable broth
- 2 tablespoons minced garlic
- 1 teaspoon dried oregano
- ½ teaspoon crushed red pepper flakes
- 1 can (14 ounces) crushed tomatoes (for a smoky flavor use fire-roasted)
- ½ cup pitted Kalamata olives or other black olives, sliced
- 2 tablespoons capers
- 1 tablespoon nutritional yeast flakes, plus additional for garnishing
- ⅓ cup chopped fresh basil, lightly packed
- 3 tablespoons chopped fresh parsley, lightly packed
- Sea salt
- Freshly ground black pepper

1. To cook the pasta, fill a large saucepan or soup pot two-thirds full with water and add a little salt to the water if desired. Bring to a boil over medium-high heat.

2. Add the pasta and cook, stirring occasionally, according to the package instructions or until tender. Reserve ¼ cup of the pasta water. Drain the pasta in a colander.

3. While the pasta is cooking, make the sauce. Put the onion, bell pepper, and oil (for an oil-free version use vegetable broth) in a large cast iron or nonstick skillet and cook over medium heat, stirring occasionally, for 5 minutes. Add the garlic, oregano, and red pepper flakes, and cook, stirring occasionally, for 2 to 3 minutes, until the vegetables are tender.

4. Add the reserved pasta water, crushed tomatoes, olives, capers, and nutritional yeast, and cook, stirring occasionally, for 2 minutes. Add the basil and parsley, and cook for 1 minute longer to blend the flavors. Remove from the heat. Season with salt and pepper to taste.

5. Add the cooked pasta and gently toss to combine. Garnish individual servings with nutritional yeast as desired. Serve hot.

Pita Pizza Party

MAKES 4 SERVING

Forget ordering from your local pizza shop--why not stay home and make pizza in your oven instead? For ease, forego making your own pizza dough, and instead use pita breads, which are ideal for making individual pizzas. These Mediterranean-style pita pizzas can be served up for dinner, lunch, or as a snack.

- 4 (6-inch) pita breads
- 12 tablespoons jarred marinara sauce
- 1 cup coarsely chopped baby spinach, lightly packed
- 6 tablespoons sliced or diced red or yellow onion
- 6 tablespoons sliced or diced red or orange bell pepper
- 8 artichoke hearts, each heart quartered, or 4 button or cremini mushrooms, thinly sliced
- 1 cup vegan shredded mozzarella cheese or other variety, or ¾ cup Cheesy Sauce (see Bacon Cheeseburger Mac-n-Cheese in this chapter)
- 4 teaspoons nutritional yeast flakes
- Freshly ground black pepper
- Crushed red pepper flakes (optional)

1. Preheat the oven to 425 degrees F. Line a baking sheet with parchment paper or a silicone baking mat. Place the pita breads on the baking sheet.

2. To assemble each pizza, spread 3 tablespoons marinara sauce evenly over the top of the pita. Scatter 1½ tablespoons of onion, 1½ tablespoons of bell pepper, and 2 quartered artichoke hearts (or 1 sliced mushroom) over the marinara sauce. Sprinkle ¼ cup of shredded cheese (or 3 tablespoons of cheesy sauce) and 1 teaspoon of nutritional yeast over the top. Season with pepper and optional red pepper flakes to taste.

3. Bake for 8 to 10 minutes, until the pita breads are lightly browned around the edges and the cheese is melted. Cut into 4 pieces. Serve hot.

BBQ Seitan Strips

MAKES 4 SERVINGS OR 12 STRIPS

A batch of homemade seitan is patted into a baking pan, scored into rib-style strips, and then partially baked. The seitan strips are then covered on both sides with a sweet-n-spicy barbecue sauce and baked until lip-smacking-good! Serve the saucy strips as a main dish, or cut them into cubes and add to bean or grain dishes.

Sweet-n-Spicy BBQ Sauce:
- ⅔ cup ketchup
- 2 tablespoons grated yellow onion
- 2 large cloves garlic, minced
- 1½ tablespoons apple cider vinegar
- 1½ tablespoons molasses or maple syrup, or 2 tablespoon coconut sugar
- 1 tablespoon bourbon (optional)
- 1 tablespoon spicy brown or whole grain mustard
- 1½ teaspoons chili powder
- ½ teaspoon ground cumin
- ½ teaspoon ground coriander
- ½ teaspoon sea salt
- ¼ teaspoon freshly ground black pepper
- ¼ teaspoon liquid smoke (optional)
- ⅛ teaspoon cayenne or hot pepper sauce

Seitan Strips:
- 1 cup vital wheat gluten
- ¼ cup chickpea flour
- 2 tablespoons nutritional yeast flakes
- 1 teaspoon garlic powder
- 1 teaspoons onion powder
- 1 cup water
- 2 tablespoons tahini, peanut butter, or other nut or seed butter
- 1 tablespoon reduced-sodium tamari or coconut aminos

1. To make the sweet-n-spicy BBQ sauce, put all of the ingredients in a small saucepan and cook over low heat, stirring occasionally, for 8 minutes, until the BBQ sauce is hot and bubbly. Remove from the heat.

2. Preheat the oven to 350 degrees F. Lightly oil a 9-inch baking pan or mist it with cooking spray.

3. To make the seitan strips, put the vital wheat gluten, flour, nutritional yeast, garlic powder, and onion powder in a large bowl and stir to combine.

4. Put the water, tahini, and tamari in a small bowl and stir to combine.

5. Add the water mixture to the vital wheat gluten mixture and stir to combine. Using your hands, knead the mixture in the bowl for 1 to 2 minutes, until the mixture forms a smooth and pliable dough. Let the seitan mixture rest for 5 minutes.

6. Transfer the seitan mixture to the oiled baking pan. Using your hands, evenly flatten the dough to cover the bottom of the baking pan. Using a sharp knife, cut (score) the dough lengthwise into 6 strips, turn the pan a one-quarter turn, and cut widthwise through the middle of each strip, to yield 12 strips.

7. Bake for 25 minutes. Remove from the oven. Using a metal spatula, loosen the seitan from the sides and bottom of the baking pan, and then cut (score) the seitan into 12 strips again. Spread half of the sweet-n-spicy BBQ sauce over the seitan strips. Bake for 7 minutes.

8. Remove from the oven. Using a metal spatula, carefully flip over the seitan strips. Spread the remaining BBQ sauce over the top. Bake for 8 to 10 minutes longer, until the seitan strips are firm to the touch and the BBQ sauce is slightly caramelized. Let cool slightly before serving. Serve hot, at room temperature, or cold as desired.

Winter Squash with Apple-Walnut Stuffing

MAKES 4 SERVINGS

If someone tells you to "get stuffed!," it can be a good thing, especially, if they're referring to a vegetable! Winter squash halves are stuffed with a sweet and savory mixture of bread cubes, apple, aromatic vegetables, dried fruit, and walnuts, and then baked until soft. This is an excellent main dish (or side dish) to make during the fall and winter months, or as part of a holiday meal.

- 2 medium winter squash (such as acorn, carnival, delicata, or sweet dumpling)
- 4 cups whole grain bread, cut into 1-inch cubes
- 1 large apple, peeled, cored, and diced
- ½ cup diced red or yellow onion
- ½ cup diced celery
- 2 teaspoons olive oil, or ¼ cup low-sodium vegetable broth or water
- ⅓ cup coarsely chopped raw walnuts
- ¼ cup thinly sliced green onions
- ¼ cup dried cranberries or raisins
- 1½ tablespoons nutritional yeast flakes
- 1 teaspoon dried thyme
- ½ teaspoon ground cinnamon
- 1 cup low-sodium vegetable broth
- ¼ cup chopped fresh parsley, lightly packed
- Sea salt
- Freshly ground black pepper

1. Preheat the oven to 375 degrees F.

2. Cut the winter squash in half (from the stem to the bottom). Using a spoon, scoop out the seeds and discard. Put the squash halves (cut-side-up) in a 13 x 9-inch baking pan. Add a little water to the bottom of the baking pan. Bake for 15 minutes.

3. While the squash is baking, make the stuffing mixture. Place the bread cubes on a baking sheet and let sit for 15 minutes to allow them to dry out.

4. Put the apple, onion, celery, and oil (for an oil-free version use vegetable broth) in a large cast iron or nonstick skillet and cook over medium heat, stirring occasionally, for 5 minutes. Add the walnuts, green onions, parsley, cranberries, nutritional yeast, thyme, and cinnamon and cook, stirring occasionally, for 3 minutes.

5. Transfer the dry bread cubes to a large bowl. Add the apple mixture, vegetable broth, and parsley and gently stir to moisten the bread cubes. Season with salt and pepper to taste.

6. Remove the squash from the oven. Evenly dividing, fill the squash halves with the stuffing mixture. Bake for 15 to 20 minutes longer, until the squash halves are tender and the stuffing is lightly browned on top. Serve hot.

Supper-Sized Stuffed Florentine Portobellos

MAKES 4 SERVINGS

Stuffed mushrooms, commonly made with button mushrooms, are often served as an appetizer. Those bite-sized morsels provided the inspiration for these supper-worthy, stuffed portobello mushrooms. These feature a savory tofu, spinach, sun-dried tomato, and breadcrumb-based filling that's topped with shredded mozzarella cheese.

- ⅓ cup hot water
- 5 whole sun-dried tomatoes, or ⅓ cup chopped sun-dried tomato pieces
- 4 large portobello mushrooms
- ½ cup finely diced celery
- ½ cup finely diced yellow onion
- ½ cup thinly sliced green onions
- 1 tablespoon olive oil
- 8 ounces firm or extra-firm tofu
- 1½ cups coarsely chopped baby spinach or arugula, lightly packed
- 1½ tablespoons minced garlic
- 1½ teaspoons dried basil
- 1½ teaspoons dried oregano
- ¾ cup dry breadcrumbs or blanched almond flour
- 2 tablespoons nutritional yeast flakes
- 2 tablespoons chopped fresh parsley
- ½ teaspoon sea salt
- ½ teaspoon freshly ground black pepper
- ¾ cup vegan shredded mozzarella cheese

1. Put the water and sun-dried tomatoes in a small bowl. Let sit for 10 minutes to rehydrate and soften the tomatoes. Drain off the soaking liquid. If using whole sun-dried tomatoes, coarsely chop them and set aside.

2. Preheat the oven to 375 degrees F. Line a baking sheet with parchment paper or a silicone baking mat.

3. Remove the stems from the mushrooms and finely chop them. Place the mushroom caps (stem-side-up) onto the lined baking sheet.

4. To make the filling, put the chopped mushroom stems, celery, onion, green onions, and oil in a large cast iron or nonstick skillet and cook over medium-high heat, stirring occasionally, for 5 minutes. Using your fingers, crumble the tofu into the skillet, and cook, stirring occasionally, for 3 minutes.

5. Add the reserved sun-dried tomatoes, spinach, garlic, basil, and oregano, and cook, stirring occasionally, for 2 minutes. Remove from the heat. Add the breadcrumbs, nutritional yeast, parsley, salt, and pepper and stir to combine.

6. Evenly dividing, fill each mushroom cap with one-quarter of the filling mixture. Sprinkle 3 tablespoons of shredded cheese over the top of each mushroom. Bake for 22 to 25 minutes, until the mushrooms are tender. Serve hot.

Cornmeal and Pumpkin Seed Breaded Tempeh

MAKES 4 SERVINGS OR 8 PIECES

Pieces of tempeh are briefly marinated in a seasoned vegan buttermilk mixture, and then coated with a savory and slightly crunchy breading mixture that's made with cornmeal and pumpkin seeds. Serve the breaded tempeh pieces as a main dish with your favorite sides, or use them on sandwiches or salads as desired.

Seasoned Vegan Buttermilk:
- ½ cup plain soy milk or other nondairy milk
- 1 teaspoon reduced-sodium tamari
- 1 teaspoon apple cider vinegar or lemon juice
- ½ teaspoon garlic powder
- ½ teaspoon onion powder
- 2 packages (8 ounces) tempeh

Breading:
- ½ cup raw pumpkin seeds
- ½ cup medium-grind cornmeal
- 3 tablespoons nutritional yeast flakes
- 2 teaspoons dried basil
- 1½ teaspoons chili powder
- 1 teaspoon dried oregano
- ¾ teaspoon ground coriander or ground cumin
- ½ teaspoon sea salt
- ¼ teaspoon freshly ground black pepper

1. To make the seasoned vegan buttermilk, put all of the ingredients (except tempeh) in a 9 x 13-inch baking pan and whisk to combine. Let sit for 5 minutes to thicken.

2. Cut each package of tempeh into 4 pieces. Using a fork, pierce each piece of tempeh several times along its length, flip over each piece, and pierce the other side in the same manner.

3. Add the tempeh pieces to the buttermilk mixture and flip over each piece to evenly coat on all sides. Place in the refrigerator to marinate for 1 hour or more as desired.

4. Preheat the oven to 400 degrees F. Line a baking sheet with parchment paper or a silicone baking mat.

5. To make the breading, put all of the ingredients in a food processor and process for 1 to 2 minutes, until the pumpkin seeds are finely ground.

6. Transfer the breading mixture to a large plate. One at a time, place the tempeh pieces into the breading mixture, pressing down slightly and flipping over as needed to evenly coat the slices on all sides.

7. Place the breaded tempeh pieces on the lined baking sheet, spacing them 2 inches apart. Bake for 20 minutes. Remove from the oven. Flip over the tempeh pieces with a fork. Bake for 15 to 20 minutes longer, until the breading is lightly browned and crispy. Serve hot.

Coconut-Crusted Cutlets with Sweet Thai Chili Sauce

MAKES 4 SERVINGS OR 8 CUTLETS

Coconut shrimp was the inspiration for this recipe, in which pieces of tofu are pressed, marinated, and then covered in a shredded coconut-enhanced coating. Serve the baked cutlets with the sweet Thai chili sauce, alongside stir-fried vegetables and cooked rice, for a stay-at-home, restaurant-style meal.

Marinade:
- 1 pound firm or extra-firm tofu
- 3 tablespoons warm water
- 1 tablespoon ground flaxseeds or flaxseed meal
- 2 tablespoons reduced-sodium tamari
- 1 tablespoon minced garlic
- 1 tablespoon peeled and grated fresh ginger

Sweet Thai Chili Sauce:
- 1 cup coconut water
- ½ cup unbleached cane sugar
- ⅓ cup rice vinegar or apple cider vinegar
- 1½ tablespoons minced garlic
- 1½ tablespoons peeled and grated fresh ginger
- 2 tablespoons cold water
- 1 tablespoon cornstarch
- 1½ teaspoons crushed red pepper flakes
- 1½ teaspoons hot pepper sauce
- ½ teaspoon sea salt

Breading:
- ⅔ cup unsweetened shredded dried coconut
- ⅓ cup blanched almond flour
- 2 tablespoons coconut sugar or unbleached cane sugar
- ½ teaspoon garlic powder
- ½ teaspoon sea salt
- ¼ teaspoon freshly ground black pepper

1. To prep the tofu, squeeze the block of tofu over the sink to remove the excess water. Place the tofu in a colander in the sink, cover with a plate, place a heavy can (or other weight) on top of the plate, and let the tofu press for 20 minutes.

2. Cut the pressed tofu lengthwise into 8 slices. Using a fork, pierce each piece of tofu several times along its length, flip over each piece, and pierce the other side in the same manner.

3. To make the marinade, put the water and flaxseeds in a 9-inch baking pan and whisk to combine. Let sit for 10 minutes to thicken into a gel.

4. Add the tamari, garlic, and ginger and whisk to combine. Add the tofu pieces and flip over each piece to evenly coat on all sides. Place in the refrigerator to marinate for 1 hour or more as desired.

5. To make the sweet Thai chili sauce, put the coconut water, sugar, vinegar, garlic, and ginger in a small saucepan and stir to combine. Bring to a boil over high heat. Decrease the heat to medium and cook, stirring occasionally, for 3 minutes.

6. Put the cold water and cornstarch in a small bowl and stir to combine. Add the cornstarch mixture, red pepper flakes, hot pepper sauce, and salt to the saucepan and cook, whisking occasionally, for 1 to 2 minutes, until the sauce thickens. Remove from the heat. Let cool slightly.

7. Preheat the oven to 400 degrees F. Line a baking sheet with parchment paper or a silicone baking mat.

8. To make the breading, put all of the ingredients on a large plate and toss with your fingers to combine. One at a time, place the tofu slices into the breading mixture, pressing down slightly and flipping over as needed to evenly coat the slices on all sides.

9. Place the breaded tofu slices on the lined baking sheet, spacing them 2 inches apart. Bake for 25 minutes. Remove from the oven. Flip over the tofu slices with a fork. Bake for 15 to 20 minutes longer, until the breading is golden brown and crispy. Serve hot with the sweet Thai chili sauce as desired.

Hot Tamale Pie

MAKES 4 SERVINGS

Hot and spicy and oh-so-yummy! This tamale pie features a veggie and bean chili-like filling that's covered with a cornbread topping. This Southwestern-style casserole makes for a hearty and filling meal any day of the week.

Chili Filling:
- ½ cup water
- ½ cup diced red or yellow onion
- ½ cup diced orange or red bell pepper
- ½ cup frozen cut corn
- ½ cup diced sweet potato
- ½ cup diced zucchini
- 1 jalapeño chile, seeded and finely sliced
- 1½ tablespoons minced garlic
- 2 teaspoons chili powder
- 1 teaspoon dried oregano
- ½ teaspoon dried ground cumin
- ½ teaspoon ground coriander
- ¼ teaspoon chipotle chili powder or cayenne
- 1 can (14 ounces) crushed tomatoes (for a smoky flavor use fire-roasted with green chiles)
- 1 can (15 ounces) beans (such as black beans, kidney beans, pinto beans, or mixed beans), drained and rinsed
- ¼ cup chopped fresh cilantro or parsley, lightly packed
- Sea salt
- Freshly ground black pepper

Cornbread Topping:
- ⅔ cup medium-grind cornmeal
- ½ cup whole wheat pastry flour
- 2 teaspoons aluminum-free baking powder
- ¼ teaspoon sea salt
- ¾ cup plain nondairy milk
- 1½ tablespoons sunflower oil or other oil

1. Preheat the oven to 400 degrees F. Lightly oil a 9-inch baking pan or mist it with cooking spray.

2. To make the chili filling, put the water, onion, bell pepper, corn, sweet potato, zucchini, jalapeño chile, and garlic in a large cast iron or nonstick skillet and cook over medium heat, stirring occasionally, for 7 minutes. Add the chili powder, oregano, cumin, coriander,

and chipotle chili powder and cook, stirring occasionally, for 2 to 3 minutes, until the vegetables are tender and the water has evaporated. Remove from the heat.

3.   Add the crushed tomatoes, beans, and cilantro, and stir to combine. Season with salt and pepper to taste. Transfer the chili filling to the oiled baking pan.

4.   To make the cornbread topping, put the cornmeal, flour, baking powder, and salt in a small bowl and whisk to combine. Add the milk and oil and whisk until smooth. Pour the cornbread topping over the chili filling and smooth the top with a spatula.

5.   Bake for 20 to 25 minutes, until the cornbread topping is lightly browned on top. Let sit for 5 minutes before serving. Serve hot.

CHAPTER 22

Happy Endings–Sweet Treats and Desserts

Who doesn't like a happy ending? Whether it's at the end of a sappy story or sexual escapade, most of us like when things have a happy ending. And, in this case, it means a happy ending in the form of a something to satisfy your sweet tooth. Flip through the pages ahead and you'll find no-bake, baked, poached, and chilled recipes for bite-sized sweet treats, puddings, cookies, cakes, and other delectable desserts. Enjoy sharing these lovingly-made indulgences with those you love!

Raw Fruity Delights

MAKES 2 SERVINGS

When it comes to serving fresh fruit, often it's best to keep the preparation and presentation simple. You'll be pleasantly surprised by the flavor of this lusciously smooth purée that's made by blending together orange juice-soaked dates along with mango and nectarines. While this purée tastes great by itself, it tastes even better and is more eye-catching when topped with berries, kiwi, and pomegranate seeds.

- ¼ cup orange juice
- 4 pitted soft dates
- 2 nectarines or peaches, peeled and diced
- 1 mango, peeled, pitted, and diced
- ¾ cup whole berries (such as blueberries, blackberries, or raspberries), or ⅔ cup sliced strawberries
- 1 kiwi, peeled, cut into quarters lengthwise, and thinly sliced
- ¼ cup pomegranate seeds, or 2 tablespoons goji berries

1. Put the orange juice and dates in a small bowl. Let sit for 15 minutes to plump the dates.

2. Put the orange juice mixture in a food processor and process for 30 seconds. Add the nectarines and mango and process until smooth. Scrape down the sides of the container with a spatula.

3. Transfer the mixture to a medium bowl. Scatter the berries, kiwi, and pomegranate seeds over the top. Serve immediately.

Spiked Dark Chocolate Truffles

MAKES 4 SERVINGS OR 12 TRUFFLES

Transform store-bought dark chocolate bars (or chocolate chips) into a batch of vegan truffles with very little effort. Just chop it up, melt it with some coconut milk, coconut oil, a bit of booze, and flavorings, and then roll the chilled chocolatey mix in your favorite topping. Voilà - you have homemade truffles that literally melt in your mouth!

- 2 bars (3 ounces and at least 70% dark chocolate) vegan dark chocolate bars, coarsely chopped, or 1 cup vegan chocolate chips
- ¼ cup canned coconut milk (full-fat and not the lite variety)
- 2 tablespoons coconut oil
- 2 tablespoons red wine of choice, or 1 tablespoon rum, whiskey, Amaretto, coffee liqueur, or other liquor or liqueur of choice
- ½ teaspoon vanilla extract
- Pinch of sea salt
- Cacao powder or unsweetened cocoa powder for rolling the truffles
- Toppings options: additional cacao powder, cacao nibs, powdered sugar, finely ground nuts, or unsweetened shredded dried coconut

---

1. Put the chopped chocolate bar, coconut milk, oil, wine, vanilla extract, and pinch of salt in a small bowl and put in the microwave for 1 to 2 minutes to melt the chocolate. Alternatively, put them in a double boiler over medium-low heat until the chocolate is melted.

2. Transfer the chocolate mixture to a 8-inch baking pan. Refrigerate for 1 hour or until firm and set, but still pliable.

3. Portion the chocolate mixture using a 1-inch ice-cream scoop or a tablespoonful for each truffle and place on a large plate lined with parchment or wax paper. Lightly coat hands with the cacao powder, roll each portion into a ball, and then place the truffles back on the plate. Refrigerate for 30 minutes.

4. Roll each truffle in topping of choice as desired. Place the coated truffles on another large plate lined with parchment or wax paper. Refrigerate the truffles for 15 minutes before serving. Store in an airtight container in the refrigerator.

Variation: Vary the flavor of the truffles, by also adding ¼ teaspoon of ground spices (such as cinnamon, cardamom, or cayenne) or flavoring extract (such as almond, coconut, or peppermint) to the melted chocolate mixture.

Cherry Amaretto Chia Seed Pudding
MAKES 2 SERVINGS

This no-cooking-required recipe has energy-enhancing chia seeds to thank for its pudding-like consistency. Also, you'll be pleasantly surprised by how much the combo of cherries, almonds, coconut milk, and a little maca powder replicates the flavor of Cherry Amaretto ice cream. This tasty treat can be served for dessert, breakfast, or as a snack.

- 1½ cups fresh or frozen sweet or sour cherries, pitted
- 1 cup plain or vanilla coconut milk beverage
- 6 tablespoons raw sliced almonds
- 2 tablespoons agave nectar, maple syrup, or coconut sugar
- 2 teaspoons maca powder
- 1 teaspoon vanilla extract
- ½ teaspoon almond extract, or 2 tablespoons Amaretto
- 3 tablespoons chia seeds

1. Coarsely chop ½ cup of cherries. Transfer them to a small bowl and refrigerate until serving.

2. Put the remaining 1 cup of cherries, milk, 4 tablespoons of sliced almonds, agave nectar, maca powder, vanilla extract, and almond extract in a blender and process until smooth. Scrape down the sides of the container with a spatula. Add the chia seeds and process for 15 seconds.

3. Transfer the mixture to a small bowl and refrigerate for 1 hour, until the chia seeds swell and thicken the mixture to a pudding-like consistency.

4. Before serving, whisk the mixture to break up any clumps of chia seeds. Evenly divide the mixture between two bowls. Top each serving with ¼ cup of the reserved chopped cherries and 1 tablespoon of sliced almonds.

Raspberry Chia Seed Pudding: Replace the cherries with 1½ cups fresh or frozen raspberries, and omit the almond extract.

Amazing Avocado-Chocolate Mousse
MAKES 2 SERVINGS

When you taste this rich and creamy mousse, not only will you be amazed that it's vegan, but even more so, by what's in it! At first, you might think that there's some strange bedfellows in this recipe, but each one brings something delightful to the mix. Serve it plain, or topped with your choice of berries, cacao nibs or chopped chocolate, and/or Whipped Coconut Cream (see recipe in this chapter).

- 1 medium banana, broken into 4 pieces
- 1 avocado, diced
- ¼ cup almond butter, peanut butter, or other nut or seed butter
- ¼ cup cacao powder or unsweetened cocoa powder
- 2 teaspoons maca powder (optional)
- 1 teaspoon vanilla extract
- Pinch of sea salt

1. Put all of the ingredients in a food processor and process until smooth. Scrape down the sides of the container with a spatula and process for 15 seconds.

2. Transfer the mixture to a small bowl. Serve immediately or refrigerate as desired. Evenly divide the mixture between two bowls. Serve plain or with toppings of choice.

Filled Figs Three Way

EACH VERSION MAKES 4 SERVINGS OR 12 FILLED FIGS

To truly appreciate their inner beauty, split open fresh figs at the top, and then gently pull them open to reveal their succulent interior. While you could savor them right now, why not fill that open cavity with something scrumptious? Because sometimes it's hard to decide, three different filling options are presented below, and whichever one you choose will be simply elegant and delicious!

- Use 12 fresh figs for each filling option

Mock Marzipan:
- 1¼ cups raw sliced almonds
- ¾ cup powdered sugar
- 1 tablespoon agave nectar
- 1 tablespoon water
- ¾ teaspoon vanilla extract
- ¼ teaspoon almond extract

Strawberry Cream Cheese and Pistachio:
- ¾ cup Strawberry-Cashew Cream Cheese Spread (see recipe in Morning Quickies)

- 12 fresh figs
- 2 to 3 tablespoons finely chopped raw or roasted pistachios

Coconut Cream Pie:
- ¾ cup Whipped Coconut Cream (see recipe in this chapter)
- 12 fresh figs
- 3 tablespoons unsweetened shredded dried coconut, raw or lightly toasted

1. To prep each fig, cut off the stem and discard. Cut an "X" into fig (from the stem toward the bottom and without cutting all the way through), and then gently open the top portion of the fig (like a flower starting to open). Place the figs on a large plate or platter and fill as desired.

2. If making the marzipan filling, reserve 12 sliced almonds for garnish. Put the remaining almonds and other ingredients (except figs) in a food processor and process until a smooth paste. Transfer to a small bowl and refrigerate for 15 minutes. Using your hands, roll 1 tablespoon portions into a log. Put 1 log into the center of each fig, and then stick one reserved sliced almond into the center of each log.

3. If making the strawberry cream cheese filling, put the mixture into a pastry bag fitted with a star tip. Alternatively, put the mixture into a small zipper-lock bag, seal the bag, and then snip off one of the bottom corners of the bag with scissors. Decoratively pipe approximately 1 tablespoon of the mixture into the center of each fig. Garnish each filled fig with chopped pistachios as desired.

4. If making the coconut cream filling, put the mixture into a pastry bag fitted with a star tip. Alternatively, put the mixture into a small zipper-lock bag, seal the bag, and then snip off one of the bottom corners of the bag with scissors. Decoratively pipe approximately 1 tablespoon of the mixture into the center of each fig. Garnish each filled fig with shredded coconut as desired.

Variation: When fresh figs aren't available, you can replace them with dried figs or pitted medjool dates, that are cut in half lengthwise. But only use half of the amount of filling to sandwich the two halves together.

Vanilla- Infused Banana Ice Cream and Partners
MAKES 2 SERVINGS

Using a food processor or a blender with a tamper attachment, you can transform frozen bananas, nondairy milk, and some vanilla extract into a lusciously-creamy, soft serve-style ice cream. Enjoy this ice cream right away as is, or top it as desired with additional chopped fruit or nuts. This recipe is highly adaptable, and check out the Variations below for additional flavor options.

- 2 very ripe large bananas, broken into 4 pieces and frozen
- ¼ cup plain or vanilla coconut milk beverage or other nondairy milk
- 1½ teaspoons vanilla extract

1. Put the bananas, milk, and vanilla extract in a food processor (or a blender with a tamper attachment) and process until smooth. Scrape down the sides of the container with a spatula and process for 15 seconds. Serve immediately.

Variation: To make an over-the-top sundae, top the ice cream with chopped fruits and nuts, and some After Dark Chocolate Sauce and Whipped Coconut Cream (see recipes in this chapter).

Maple-Walnut Banana Ice Cream: Replace the coconut milk with 2½ tablespoons almond milk and 1½ tablespoons maple syrup. Stir ⅓ cup toasted and coarsely chopped walnuts into the finished ice cream.

Chocolate, Peanut Butter, and Banana Ice Cream: Decrease the amount of coconut milk to 2½ tablespoons. Add 3 tablespoons peanut butter and 3 tablespoons cacao powder or unsweetened cocoa powder.

Berry-Banana Ice Cream: Add 1 cup fresh blueberries, raspberries, or sliced strawberries, or 1 cup frozen berries (do not thaw).

Pineapple-Banana Sherbet: Omit the vanilla extract. Add 1 cup canned or frozen pineapple chunks.

Whipped Coconut Cream

MAKES 1½ CUPS

Chilling cans of coconut milk (you can't use the lite variety) in the refrigerator overnight will make it separate, and the thick, coconut cream will congeal at the top of the can while the liquidy coconut water will remain on the bottom. Miraculously, the thick coconut cream portion can be blended to create a fluffy, nondairy whipped topping. Serve as a topping for your favorite desserts or fresh berries, or parts of your lover's body... if you're feeling naughty!

- 2 cans (14 ounces) coconut milk (full-fat and not the lite variety), refrigerated overnight
- ⅓ cup powdered sugar
- 1½ teaspoons vanilla extract

1. Chill a large bowl and electric mixer beaters in the freezer for 20 minutes.

2. Carefully open the chilled coconut milk. Using a spoon, skim the thick, white coconut cream from the top of each can, avoiding the thin watery liquid in the bottom of the can (or it won't whip properly), and put the coconut cream in the chilled bowl. The remaining watery liquid can be used in smoothies or discarded.

3. Beat the coconut cream with an electric mixer for 2 to 3 minutes, until soft peaks form.

4. Add the sugar and vanilla extract and beat for 1 minute. Store in an airtight container in the refrigerator.

Variation: For an easier preparation, replace the two cans of chilled coconut milk with 1 can (14 ounces) coconut cream, refrigerated overnight. You can find coconut cream alongside canned coconut milk in most grocery stores.

After Dark Chocolate Sauce and Fondue-for-Two

MAKES 1⅔ CUPS SAUCE (⅓ CUP SERVING AS A SAUCE)

To create this velvety-rich and chocolaty sauce, nondairy milk, sweetener of choice, and vanilla extract are combined with both cacao powder and vegan chocolate chips (or chopped dark chocolate bars). If you want it a bit boozy, then add the optional liqueur. Or if you like it spicy, then add the suggested cinnamon or cayenne. You can use the finished chocolate sauce hot or warm as a topping for desserts or nondairy ice cream, or chill to solidify the sauce for use as a body paint for licking off your lover. Also, check out the Variation below for how to serve it fondue-style as a romantic treat for two!

- **After Dark Chocolate Sauce:**
- 1¼ cups plain or vanilla soy milk or other nondairy milk
- ¼ cup cacao powder or unsweetened cocoa powder
- 2 tablespoon agave nectar, maple syrup, or unbleached cane sugar
- Pinch of sea salt
- 1 cup vegan chocolate chips, or 2 bars (3 ounces and at least 70% dark chocolate) vegan dark chocolate bars, coarsely chopped
- 1½ teaspoons vanilla extract
- 1 tablespoons liqueur or liquor of choice (such as cherry, orange, coffee, rum, or bourbon) (optional)
- ¼ teaspoon ground cinnamon or cayenne (optional)

1. Put the milk, cacao powder, agave nectar, and pinch of salt in a small saucepan and whisk to combine. Cook the mixture over medium heat, whisking occasionally, for 2 to 3 minutes, until the mixture just begins to bowl.

2. Remove from the heat. Add the chocolate chips and vanilla and whisk until the chocolate chips are completely melted. If desired, whisk in the optional liqueur or liquor and/or cinnamon or cayenne. Serve hot, warm, or at room temperature as desired. Store in an airtight container in the refrigerator. Chilling the sauce will thicken it to a ganache-like consistency.

Fondue-for Two: Serve the warm After Dark Chocolate Sauce with your choice of things for dipping into it. Here are some suggestions: whole strawberries or raspberries, whole cherries, whole seedless grapes, thick slices of banana, pineapple chunks, pretzels, or large cubes of cake.

Cherries Jubilee

MAKES 2 CUPS OR 4 SERVINGS

Flambéed desserts are often dramatically prepared table-side in restaurants. But you can also successfully and safely make them at home as well, and before you start, check out the safety tips that follow this recipe. Cherries Jubilee is a simple, yet show-stopping dessert, which is made by briefly cooking cherries in a lemon-flavored syrup, and the tender cherries are then doused with a bit of booze and dramatically flambéed. Serve as a topping for nondairy ice cream, pieces of cake, or other desserts as desired.

- 1 pound fresh or frozen sweet or sour cherries, pitted
- ⅓ cup unbleached cane sugar
- 2 tablespoons nonhydrogenated vegan butter
- Zest and Juice of ½ a lemon
- ¼ cup liqueur or liquor of choice (such as brandy, Amaretto, Kirsch, or orange liqueur)

1. Put the cherries and sugar in a large cast iron or nonstick skillet and cook over medium-high heat, stirring occasionally, for 5 to 7 minutes, until the sugar is fully dissolved and the cherries are soft.

2. Add the vegan butter and lemon zest and juice and cook, stirring constantly, for 1 minute, until the vegan butter is melted.

3. Using a long-handled metal spoon, stir in the liquor/liqueur of choice. Carefully light a long match and hold it to the cherry mixture to flambé (ignite) the alcohol vapors (for a dramatic effect, do this with the lights dimmed). When the flame has subsided to a small blue flame, gently stir the mixture to cook off any residual alcohol vapors in the skillet. Remove from the heat. Serve hot or warm as desired.

Tips: When preparing any flambéed dish, be very careful to avoid getting burned, or worse yet, causing a fire! Avoid wearing long (or hanging) sleeves, be cautious of dangling or long hair, and if you're wearing a tie, then tuck it in. After igniting the alcohol, wait for the big flame to die down to a small blue flame, before stirring the dish with a metal spoon to expose any residual alcohol to the flame. Flambéing helps to reduce the strong alcohol flavor and caramelizes sugars, as well as makes for an entertaining presentation. Just in case something goes awry, keep an appropriate-sized lid nearby (to quickly snuff out the flames), and know where your fire extinguisher is located.

Mulled Wine Poached Pears
MAKES 4 SERVINGS

This is an elegant, yet simple to make dessert, which is perfect for a fall or winter evening. Large, firm pears are peeled and poached in a robustly-spiced red wine mixture until tender. Serve the poached pears topped with some of the poaching liquid, as well as with a dollop or two of vanilla nondairy yogurt if desired.

- ½ of a large orange
- 2 cups red wine of choice (such as Burgundy, Merlot, or Cabernet Sauvignon)
- ¼ cup maple syrup or light brown sugar
- 1 (3-inch) cinnamon stick
- 3 whole allspice, or ¼ teaspoon ground allspice
- 3 whole cloves
- 4 large pears (such as Bosc, Comice, or D'Anjou)
- Vanilla nondairy yogurt (optional)

1. Using a vegetable peeler, remove 2 to 3 long strips of the zest from the orange half, and place them in a large saucepan. Add the wine, maple syrup, cinnamon stick, allspice, and cloves. Bring to a boil over high heat. Cover, decrease the heat to low, and simmer for 5 minutes.

2. While the wine mixture is cooking, peel the pears, but leave the stems intact. Place the pears in the wine mixture and tilt the pears on their sides to submerge them as much as possible. Cover and simmer for 15 to 20 minutes, turning the pears over every 5 minutes to ensure even coloring and cooking, until the pears are tender and easily pierced with the tip of a sharp knife.

3. Remove from the heat and uncover the saucepan. Let the pears cool for 15 minutes in the poaching liquid. Using a slotted spoon, transfer the pears to a large plate or platter and set aside. Also using the slotted spoon, remove the orange peel, cinnamon stick, and whole allspice and cloves, and discard them.

4. Bring the poaching liquid to a boil over medium heat. Cook the poaching liquid for 10 to 15 minutes, until the liquid is reduced by half and thickens into a syrup-like consistency. Serve the pears at room temperature. Drizzle a little of the reduced poaching liquid over the top of each pear before serving, and also top with dollops of vanilla nondairy yogurt if desired.

Sugar-n-Spice-Kissed Cookies

MAKES 30 COOKIES

Do you find the smell of cinnamon to be quite the aphrodisiac? Then the aroma of these cinnamon-sugar-coated cookies baking in the oven will undoubtedly be irresistible! They're also made with a combination of almond flour and coconut oil, which gives them a melt-in-your-mouth texture.

- 2½ tablespoons water
- 1 teaspoon chia seeds
- 2 tablespoons plus ⅔ cup unbleached cane sugar
- 2 teaspoons ground cinnamon
- 3 cups blanched almond flour
- ¾ teaspoon baking soda
- ¼ teaspoon sea salt
- 4 tablespoons melted coconut oil
- 1½ tablespoons vanilla extract

1. Preheat the oven to 350 degrees F. Line two baking sheets with parchment paper or silicone baking mats.

2. Put the water and chia seeds in a small bowl and stir to combine. Let sit for 10 minutes to thicken into a gel.

3. Put 2 tablespoons of sugar and cinnamon in a small bowl and stir to combine.

4. Put the remaining ¾ cup of sugar, almond flour, baking soda, and salt in a large bowl and stir to combine. Add the chia seed mixture, oil, and vanilla extract and use a fork to work them into the flour mixture to form a soft cookie dough.

5. Using your hands, roll the dough into 1-inch balls. Roll each ball in the cinnamon-sugar mixture to evenly coat on all sides. Place the balls on the lined baking sheets, spacing them 2 inches apart. Using a measuring cup or glass, slightly flatten each ball.

6. Bake for 10 to 12 minutes, until the cookies are set on top and lightly browned on the bottom and around the edges. Let cool completely on the baking sheets. Store in an airtight container at room temperature.

Pine Nut Sugary-Kiss Cookies: To the finished cookie dough, add ½ cup toasted pine nuts and 1 teaspoon ground fennel seed and stir to combine. Shape the dough into 1-inch balls, and roll them in unbleached sugar (don't add cinnamon).

Making Whoopie Pies

MAKES 12 SANDWICH COOKIES

Have you heard of whoopie pies? Well, they're just the yummiest sandwich cookies ever! Envision this - two dark chocolate, cake-like cookies are baked and cooled, and then sandwiched together with a creamy buttercream-style frosting - that's how you make a whoopie pie.

Cookies:
- 1 cup whole wheat pastry flour
- 6 tablespoons cacao powder or unsweetened cocoa powder
- ½ teaspoon baking soda
- ¼ teaspoon aluminum-free baking powder
- ¼ teaspoon sea salt
- ½ cup light brown sugar, lightly packed
- ¼ cup nonhydrogenated vegan butter
- ¼ cup plain or vanilla nondairy yogurt
- ¼ cup plain or chocolate nondairy milk
- ½ teaspoon vanilla extract

Buttercream Frosting:
- 1¼ cups powdered sugar
- 2 tablespoons nonhydrogenated vegan butter
- 1½ tablespoons plain nondairy milk
- 1 teaspoon vanilla extract

1. Preheat the oven to 350 degrees F. Line two baking sheets with parchment paper or silicone baking mats.

2. To make the cookies, put the flour, cacao powder, baking soda, baking powder, and salt in a medium bowl and whisk to combine.

3. Put the sugar, vegan butter, yogurt, milk, and vanilla extract in the bowl of an electric mixer and beat for 1 minute. Add the and reserved flour mixture and beat for 1 minute, until the mixture forms a thick batter.

4. Portion the batter on to the lined baking sheets using a 1-inch ice cream scoop or 1 level tablespoon per cookie, spacing them 2 inches apart (12 cookies per baking sheet). Slightly flatten each portion with your fingers.

5. Bake for 10 minutes, until the cookies are set on top (they will be soft). Let cool completely on the baking sheets.

6. While the cookies are cooling, make the buttercream frosting. Put all of the ingredients in the bowl of an electric mixer and beat for 2 to 3 minutes, until the frosting is light and fluffy.

7. To assemble each whoopie pie, place 1 tablespoon of the buttercream frosting on the bottom of one cookie, place another cookie (bottom-side-in) on top, and gently press the cookies together. Repeat the assembly procedure with the remaining cookies and buttercream frosting. Store in an airtight container in the refrigerator.

Vegan Berry Cheesecake

MAKES 1 (8-INCH) CHEESECAKE OR 8 SERVINGS

For this vegan and gluten-free cheesecake, almond flour, brown sugar, and melted vegan butter are used to make the crust, and vegan cream cheese and silken tofu are used in its creamy filling. To elevate its presentation, the baked and cooled cheesecake is adorned with a berry topping.

Crust:
- 1½ cups blanched almond flour
- ¼ cup light brown sugar, lightly packed
- 2 tablespoons nonhydrogenated vegan butter

Filling:
- 1 package (12 ounces) extra-firm silken tofu
- 2 containers (8 ounces) vegan cream cheese
- ⅔ cup unbleached cane sugar
- ¼ cup cornstarch
- Zest and juice of 1 lemon
- 1½ tablespoons vanilla extract

Topping:
- 1 pint fresh berries (such as blackberries, blueberries, raspberries, or sliced strawberries)
- 2 tablespoons unbleached cane sugar
- 4 tablespoons water
- 1½ teaspoons cornstarch

1. Preheat the oven to 350 degrees F. Lightly oil a 8-inch springform pan or mist it with cooking spray.

2. To make the crust, put all of the ingredients in a food processor and process for 1 minute. Transfer the crust mixture to the oiled springform pan. Using your hands, evenly flatten the mixture to cover the bottom of the pan. Bake for 8 minutes. Remove from the oven. Let cool for 5 minutes.

3. To make the filling, put all of the ingredients in a food processor and process until smooth. Scrape down the sides of the container with a spatula and process for 15 seconds. Transfer the filling mixture to the pre-baked crust and smooth the top with a spatula.

4. Place the springform pan on a baking sheet. Bake for 45 to 50 minutes, until the filling is set. Let cool for 30 minutes. Loosen the sides of the cheesecake from the pan with a knife. Place in the refrigerator to chill for 2 hours or more.

5. To make the topping, put the berries, sugar, and 2 tablespoons of water in a small saucepan and cook over medium heat, stirring occasionally, for 3 minutes. Put the remaining 2 tablespoons of water and cornstarch in a small bowl and whisk to combine. Add the cornstarch mixture to the saucepan and cook, whisking occasionally, for 1 to 2 minutes, until the topping thickens. Remove from the heat. Let cool for 10 minutes. Spoon the topping mixture over the cheesecake and refrigerate as desired.

6. Before serving, loosen the sides of the cheesecake from the pan with a knife, and remove the outer ring of the springform pan. Dip a sharp knife in warm water and wipe on a paper towel before cutting into 8 pieces. Store the cheesecake (covered) in the refrigerator.

Vanilla Pound Cake

MAKES 1 (8 X 4 X 2½-INCH) CAKE OR 8 SERVINGS

Vanilla lovers, this dense pound cake recipe is for you, as it's made with lots of vanilla-flavored ingredients. Also, rather than adding tons of oil, nondairy yogurt (or silken tofu) is used to give this low-fat pound cake a moist and tender crumb. Serve it plain, with a light dusting of powdered sugar, with a side of berries, or topped with Cherries Jubilee (see recipe in this chapter).

- 1 ⅔ cups unbleached all-purpose flour or whole wheat pastry flour
- ⅔ cup unbleached cane sugar
- 1 teaspoon baking soda
- ¼ teaspoon aluminum-free baking powder
- ¼ teaspoon sea salt
- ¾ cup vanilla nondairy milk
- 1 container (6 ounces) vanilla nondairy yogurt, or ½ cup extra-firm silken tofu, puréed
- 1 tablespoon sunflower oil or other oil
- 1 tablespoon vanilla extract

1. Preheat the oven to 350 degrees F. Lightly oil a 8 x 4 x 2½-inch loaf pan or mist it with cooking spray.

2. Put the flour, sugar, baking soda, baking powder, and salt in a large bowl and whisk to combine.

3. Put the milk, yogurt, oil, and vanilla extract in a small bowl and whisk to combine. Add the milk mixture to the flour mixture and whisk to combine.

4. Transfer the batter to the oiled loaf pan and smooth the top with the back of a spatula.

5. Bake for 30 to 35 minutes, until a toothpick inserted in the center of the cake comes out clean. Let cool in the pan for 5 minutes.

6. Loosen the sides of the cake from the pan with a knife. Invert the pan onto a rack and let the cake release naturally from the pan. Serve warm or at room temperature. Store in an airtight container at room temperature.

Vanilla-Berry Pound Cake: Stir ½ cup fresh or frozen berries (such as blueberries, blackberries, or red raspberries) into the finished cake batter.

Lemon-Poppy Seed Pound Cake: Replace ¼ cup of the nondairy milk with the zest and juice of 1 lemon (½ tablespoon zest and ¼ cup juice). Stir 1½ tablespoons poppy seeds into the finished cake batter.

Gluten-Free Vanilla Pound Cake: Replace the unbleached all-purpose flour with 1⅔ cups gluten-free baking mix and add ½ teaspoon xanthan gum.

Devil's Food Cake with After Dark Ganache

MAKES 1 (8-INCH) CAKE OR 8 SERVINGS

This dark chocolate cake tastes is so devilishly good tasting! But, are you ready for this - it's oil-free and guilt-free as well. Through culinary alchemy, a large apple, some dried dates and prunes, cacao powder, brown sugar, and coffee are transformed into a dark chocolate-flavored purée, which adds sweetness and moisture to the cake without adding any fat. The finished cake is glazed with a layer of After Dark Chocolate Sauce and then briefly chilled to harden it into a ganache-like covering.

- 1¼ cup cold coffee
- 1 large apple, peeled, cored, and diced
- 8 pitted soft dates (preferably medjool dates)
- 8 pitted prunes
- ⅔ cup cacao powder or unsweetened cocoa powder
- ⅔ cup light brown sugar or coconut sugar
- 1⅓ cups whole wheat pastry flour
- 1 teaspoon baking soda
- ½ teaspoon aluminum-free baking powder
- ½ teaspoon sea salt
- ½ teaspoon ground cinnamon
- 1 cup warm After Dark Chocolate Sauce (see recipe in this chapter)

1. Preheat the oven to 350 degrees F. Lightly oil a 8-inch springform pan (or round cake pan) or mist it with cooking spray.

2. Put the coffee, apple, dates, prunes, cacao powder, and sugar in a medium saucepan and stir thoroughly to combine. Partially cover and cook over medium heat, stirring occasionally, for 5 to 7 minutes, until the apple is soft. Remove from the heat. Let cool for 5 minutes.

3. Transfer the coffee mixture to a food processor and process until smooth. Scrape down the sides of the container with a spatula. Add the flour, baking soda, baking powder, salt, and cinnamon and process until smooth. Scrape down the sides of the container with a spatula and process for 15 seconds.

4. Transfer the batter to the oiled pan and smooth the top with the back of a spatula.

5. Bake for 30 to 35 minutes, until a toothpick inserted in the center of the cake comes out clean. Let cool in the pan for 5 minutes.

6. Loosen the sides of the cake from the pan with a knife. If using a springform pan, remove the outer ring of the springform pan. Alternatively, if using a cake pan, invert the pan onto a rack and let the cake release naturally from the pan. Let cool completely.

7. Place the cooled cake on a plate. Slowly and evenly drizzle the warm chocolate sauce over the top of the cake and use a spatula as needed, to help cover the sides of the cake with the sauce. Place the cake in the refrigerator for 10 to 15 minutes, until the sauce hardens into a ganache-like consistency.

8. Let the cake sit at room temperature for 3 minutes before cutting. Dip a sharp knife in warm water and wipe on a paper towel before cutting into 8 pieces. Store the cake (covered) in the refrigerator.